Eat!

Rediscover Your Best Natural Relationship with Food

LINDA R. HARPER, PH.D.
Foreword by THOMAS MOORE

CAP
Publishing

Copyright © 2014 by Linda R. Harper

ISBN-13 (eBook): 978-0-9913340-5-6
ISBN-13 (Trade Paperback): 978-0-9913340-4-9

This book has been designed to be a general guide and an aid to those adapting to an alternative relationship with their food. This book is not intended for use in diagnosis, treatment, or any medical application. Questions should be directed to your personal physician. This information is not warranted and no liability is assumed by the author or publisher for the recommendations, information, and suggestions promulgated. The names and identifying information of clients described in this book have been changed to protect their anonymity.

Cover design by Bri Bruce
Edited by Bri Bruce and Elizabeth Levy-Adams

WHAT READERS ARE SAYING ABOUT *EAT*

Instead of another fad diet, [Dr. Harper] introduces a method focused on teaching you how to throw away all of the diet rules and obsessions that you may not have even realized were running your life. She shows you how to look within yourself in order to find your "best self" and she gives you the tools necessary to rebuild your inner trust with food and eating. Rebuilding this trust is the key to finally achieving peace with food and becoming a "soulful" eater. I recommend this book to anyone struggling with dieting or facing a negative relationship with food; it will change how you feel about eating forever.

- Laura Graves, Empty Spoonful.com

This is a great book to read if you have problems with your weight or eating in general. . . . an astounding book in its thoughtfulness about people's relationship with food and how we should have a better relationship emotionally with what we eat. There literally are many thoughts we all should chew on (pardon the cheap pun). For someone looking for ideas to help understand your own problems with your relationship with food, this is an eye-opener.

- Richard Evans, *Fat Man Lean Man* Book Reviews

I would recommend that anyone with an unhealthy food relationship read [this book]. Eat! *is an easy, quick read that focuses on a five-step guide to healthy eating which includes: goal replacing, uncovering, informing, deciding, and experiencing.*

- Kristy Feltenberger Gillespie

I choose to read Eat! *by Dr. Linda R. Harper because I am always trying to lose ten pounds. I thought this would be another dry reading nutritional diet book. I was pleasantly surprised that it was light and easy to read. . . . Dr. Harper puts dieting into perspective by advising us to "let go of thoughts of dieting and forbidden foods." She provides you with steps that will make you look at eating in a whole new light. She wants you to enjoy your eating experience not starve yourself. . . . I recommend this book to other readers that are interested in learning about food choices and why they do not need another fad diet. They need to know there is another way to get past all the diet mumbo jumbo and starvation and begin to enjoy their meals;* Eat! *will help them do that.*

- Jan Harris

For anyone struggling with the path of dieting I recommend this book highly. . . . [The dieter] will be able to identify with the examples and will begin to transform their unhealthy relationship with themselves and food into a healthy one—and that, in the end, is Dr. Harper's goal.

- Lara Girdler, *NCReaderGirl* Book Reviews

For my father, James H. Harper, and
my mother, Mary Harper.

TABLE OF CONTENTS

FOREWORD   ◆   **1**

INTRODUCTION   ◆   **9**

AUTHOR'S NOTE   ◆   **17**

QUICK QUIZ: What Kind of Eater

  Are You?   ◆   **19**

CHAPTER I: Goal-Replacing   ◆   **23**

CHAPTER II: Uncovering   ◆   **37**

CHAPTER III: Informing   ◆   **77**

CHAPTER IV: Deciding   ◆   **101**

CHAPTER V: Experiencing   ◆   **121**

SELF-AFFIRMATIONS   ◆   **143**

CONCLUSION   ◆   **151**

AFTERWORD   ◆   **153**

ABOUT THE AUTHOR   ◆   **155**

Eat!

Rediscover Your Best Natural Relationship with Food

LINDA R. HARPER, PH.D.

FOREWORD

Food is a mystery. It looks like mere material stuff we put in our bodies for nutrition and health, and yet it does many other things as well that address out emotions, our sense of meaning, and even our spirituality. Food always has a cultural overlay or an inner life that may come from nation, region, family, or personal experience. Food may also have its mythology, its own dream life, and its religion.

You are down in the dumps about some negative development in a relationship or a situation at work, and you call up a good friend and say, "Let's have dinner." You don't say, "Let's find an empty room where we can talk." Food is part of the rite in which friends console and counsel each other.

You go to a wedding, and the joy of everyone present is translated into abundant food. You attend a funeral, and afterward everyone gathers for a meal. You go to church, and God is made present in bread and wine, which everyone eats and drinks. The celebration of Christmas, Passover, Easter, and Thanksgiving are unimaginable without special foods, and the meditating and chanting in Hindu rituals is carried on against the aromatic background of simmering spices.

You go to a hospital to visit a sick friend, and the first thing you say after looking around is, "How's the food here?" You take a long flight on an airplane, and for days you don't stop talking about how bad or surprisingly good the food was. Food has meaning as well as calories, and intuitively we know that to do anything particularly significant in life—get married, celebrate an anniversary, or just have a party—we have to do it with food.

All of these examples point to the mystery of food. Scientists and medical people talk about food as an assortment of chemicals, but we know that food is infinitely more. Why else choose Indian food one night and Italian the next? Why cook certain recipes or dress up a table or add a garnish to a special dish? Not for the chemical contributions food makes to our bodies, but for the less literal and obvious nutrients food gives to the heart and imagination. The ancient Jewish theologian Philo of Alexandria says that the word of God is food for the soul, but the reverse may also be true: Food is a way to give the soul the spiritual nourishment it requires.

It makes sense, then, that if we have trouble with food or if we are concerned about the health or look of our bodies, a diet-based, medical, materialistic, or chemical understanding of food is far too inadequate. The usual approach to dieting assumes that we and our food are elements in a materialistic world in which meaning and physical life have nothing to do with each other. But all food addresses the soul, and all food is sacramental.

When Linda Harper first showed me her manuscript, I was profoundly intrigued. It was the only attempt I had ever seen to question constructively the very idea of dieting in the usual sense and to treat food as a mysterious aspect of the soul's subtle body. Her book is full of wisdom, based on the simple idea that the human body is not divorced from meaning and emotion but is a tangible presencing of the soul.

Once we recognize that our view of human existence, and the human body in particular, has been thoroughly and negatively influenced by the materialistic philosophies of our time, then can we begin to appreciate the body's mysteries. We can see food in a different, deeper light. Myth, fantasy, metaphor, ritual and symbol all have relevance to food and therefore play a central role in our thoughts about dieting.

To delve into the soul of food, we have to consider those elements that are particular to the life of the soul: memory, fantasy, image, dream, and poetry. What is the symbolic meaning of an apple, and what precisely does a good pasta do for the soul? Do our personal memories of food affect our eating? What is the deeper meaning of fat? And what is behind our idea that being thin is good and being overweight is next to sinful?

As I think of food in my own life, I am overwhelmed by the universe of foods and ways of eating that carry my story. I can imagine writing an autobiography structured entirely according to foods I have eaten. We are what we eat, it is said, but we rarely take that wise observation deeply and seriously.

I like to bake and eat scones, preferably with strong, dark tea, a combination I can trace back to my life in Ireland in my late teens and early twenties. Fresh mozzarella cheese keeps me connected to Florence, Italy, which is meaningful to me on many levels. Whenever I eat a French Napoleon pastry, which is quite rarely, I'm taken back to a bakery in Texas and to an exciting period of my life. I have just begun to enjoy Spanish rice again now that I make it with care; when I was in high school, it was served directly out of the can. Food keeps me connected to my past, an important aspect of living a grounded, secure life.

There is also shadow in my fantasies of food— eating neuroses. I have been a reserved and contained person all of my life. I don't understand this aspect of my nature very well, but I do know that it was strengthened by growing up in a Catholic school where being quiet and invisible was considered charming. In reaction to this lifelong self-containment, I prize freedom and release in many forms, and one way I find relief is in occasional transgression of the food rules that I believe I should follow. Dr. Harper's analysis of this problematic aspect of eating is, to me, one of the most helpful aspects of her book.

Sometimes, when I am eating alone, I will indulge in foods that I have no business eating. At home, when I'm asked what I'd like to eat, I often say in jest, "Napoleons," or "Tiramisu, please." A luscious, fatty dessert to me means escape, ultimate satisfaction, parole.

All my life I have pursued many different kinds of spirituality. Once, in Ireland, I spent a weekend of self-denial on an ascetic island monastery in the middle of Lough Dergh. In penance for our sins, we retreatants stayed up all night praying and enjoyed a diet of Lough Dergh soup—hot water with salt and pepper. Ascetic spirituality often finds expression in simple and scant eating. On this island, being miserable from lack of sleep and food was considered an effective way to advance the spiritual life.

Dieting is often motivated by a spiritual fantasy of some sort. Trying to look thin has something in common with building a Gothic cathedral: they both seek transcendence in a tall, thin body that has less earth and more spirit. Both may be beautiful and worthy goals, but both can also become rigid and life-threatening. In the spiritual life, sex and food are often linked: dieting has something in common with celibacy as well. Looking closely at the spiritual fantasies hiding in our desire to diet might help show precisely where the soul might be wounded by our fervor.

A diet also has a masochistic side—self-punishment. The word "diet" originally referred to the regulation of a day, a kind of discipline, a word that sometimes refers to self-flagellation. Dieters deny themselves, and in their fantasy, they often imagine wonderful delights that are forbidden to them by their own choice. By dieting, they make themselves suffer, substituting the pleasure of self-denial for the joys of living. In the midst of a diet, it might be good to notice precisely where we are getting pleasure from pain and see if there might be a more positive source.

A diet hyperactivates the masochist in a person. The best way I know to bring soul to masochistic practices is to shift the focus of our obedience. Instead of being committed to regulations proposed by an expert on health, we could follow a deeper law and a less ego-centered philosophy. This is essentially what Dr. Harper recommends when she suggest that we leave the fantasy of dieting altogether and, instead, submit to the needs and desires of our own soul. If we eat from a deep place—not from an ego plan to be a certain kind of person but from fearless trust in the soul—our diet will take care of itself.

Another common fantasy that motivates a strenuous diet is the craving for health, which at a deeper level, often seems to be a duel with death. Health may also be a version of perfectionism, as when we commonly say that certain behaviors are healthy and others unhealthy. The word "unhealthy" sometimes sounds like a modern version of the old-fashioned "sinful." Good health is a blessing, of course, and it is a valid goal. But it is one need among many, and sometimes the soul thrives in a setting of ill health, as when a person finally discovers through a serious illness what is really important in life.

Perfectionism is an emotional complex, setting a highly spiritual ideal that we can never reach, and therefore it usually leads to pain. Its spiritual roots may not be explicit, but they are at work nonetheless. Aiming at perfection, we are trying to transcend our humanity, feel a degree of superiority, and perhaps justify our existence. Angels may be perfect, but a human being enjoys individuality and humanity by being humbly, but not humiliatingly, imperfect.

The values traditionally associated with the soul are quite different from those of the perfectionistic spirit: deep pleasure, intimacy and community, imagination, friendship, and love of all kinds. It is possible, as Dr. Harper spells out gently, to shape our eating from the deep, life-affirming place of the soul rather than in the more demanding perspective of the perfectionistic spirit.

Dieting can take soul out of our daily lives. We may take up a diet as a battle against our nature. We may spend our days suffering deprivation and self-denial. We may lose the contributions that food offers to an abundant, soulful life. We may even miss out on the soul values to be found in the fat and richness of food, in hearty family and communal eating, and in the great variety of foods and preparations available to us that make life worth living.

It's tempting to take food literally and to get caught up in counting calories and cholesterol. But one could also make a study of imagination, fantasy, and even myth—the deep narratives and images—that lie in such familiar items as fat, protein, measurement, a weighing scale, big bellies, and fatty thighs. My guess is that a researcher in the imagination of dieting would find a great deal of soul in the growing, preparing, presenting, and enjoying of food.

General reverence for life can take the special form of reverence for our food and our bodies. Trusting in the soul to shape our lives with its deep wisdom, we can eat without worry and self-consciousness. We can make cooking and eating daily arts and dining a true ritual. In this way, not only do we treat our bodies well, but we also find a way to soul through food. We might then also restore to our eating the important elements of community, family, romance, tradition, and ritual. In this way, every meal, no matter how large or small, would be an instance of caring for the soul.

I invite you to enjoy and learn from this book. It could transform the way to imagine food, the way you eat, and the way you live. It is a book both on how to bring soul to your eating habits and how to allow your eating to bring soul into the whole of life. You are what you eat, so take the lessons of this book to heart and don't eat any food that doesn't have soul.

- Thomas Moore
Author of *Care of the Soul*
www.careofthesoul.net

INTRODUCTION

Are you looking for an easy solution to a troubled relationship with food? Look no further; you already hold the answer within.

To return to the life-enriching relationship with food that you were meant to have, simply ask yourself, "What eating experience do I want now?" Allow your *best self*, that is, the deep wisdom that is already within you, to answer this question one moment at a time. Your natural and healthy relationship with food will unfold in all its brilliance and life-giving possibilities.

This *best self* is accessible to all of us; it only needs to be discovered and given a voice. Michelangelo has often been credited with saying that every block of marble contains a perfect statue that is revealed when the imprisoning walls around it are removed. Similarly, your best relationship with food emerges when you strip away the limiting thoughts that detract from the perfect moment that each eating experience offers. One such imprisoning thought is that food choices should be based on the goal of weight loss. This restrictive belief limits our natural ability to consider all the possibilities that are present to us in creating our own unique and enjoyable life with food.

This book will guide you in accessing your *best self* using one simple question: What eating experience do I want now? Let's take a closer look at this inquiry that will help you reclaim your natural relationship with food. "I" refers to your *best self*, the deepest part of you where the thoughts that you have about how to eat flow from your intuitive and natural wisdom. "Want" is your *best self*'s ability to consider the needs and desires of the whole person—body, mind, and soul—in making choices about food. "Eating experience" is what occurs when your *best self* is allowed to create unique and enjoyable interactions with food that enrich your everyday life. "Now" refers to each present moment as it comes.

And right now your *best self* is ready and eager to access the wisdom you have always had and provide an answer to this question—one moment at a time. So if it is so simple, you might ask, "Why does it feel so complicated and why does an entire book need to be written about one question?" Unfortunately we have modern society to thank for this complexity and the disconnection from our *best selves* that we experience on a regular basis when it comes to eating. For over one hundred years, our culture has promoted dieting, with the goal of losing weight, as the acceptable way to eat. I call this cultural influence SAD, an acronym that stands for Socially Acceptable Deprivation. Restricting our food choices by counting calories and grams of fat, making lists of forbidden food and measuring pounds and inches are just a few of the self- depriving actions that our society supports as the right thing to do. In reality, however, we eventually crave and indulge in the foods we label as forbidden, fail to reach our weight loss-focused goals, make unhealthy and unnatural choices, and gain back any weight that was initially lost. We then start all over again with the newest dieting fads that also continue to encourage artificial restrictions on what we allow ourselves to eat. It's an endless cycle that is created when the goal of weight loss determines food choices. Furthermore, a rule-based thought system develops that discourages you from trusting your own ability to make the best choices about eating and living.

Perhaps you can remember an enjoyable experience with food before this misdirected thinking interfered with your ability to hear the guidance of your natural wisdom. A cherished childhood memory of mine is eating ice cream one hot Saturday afternoon. With my father at the wheel and my mother at his side, I sat with my sister and my two brothers in the back seat of a newly purchased, though used, family car. Celebrating my father's raise, the new car, and good report cards, we headed out to the ice cream parlor. I remember the ice cream's sweet taste and the cool, refreshing feeling that gave my body some relief from the heat. Enjoying the moment together, my family and I laughed as our ice cream cones melted faster than we could eat them.

This event in my childhood is one example of a memorable eating experience without the influence of SAD. As a child, I was naturally thin and ate without thinking about how my food intake might affect my body. I savored the comfort I felt at the family dinner table and delighted in enjoying favorite treats with friends. Like my family ice cream outing, each eating experience created its own important part of my life, and together these experiences established a happy relationship with food that was peacefully integrated into my everyday life.

At the age of fifteen, however, I innocently embarked on my first diet. While growing up, I was encouraged to use my intelligence and I was praised for my drive for achievement. I learned that these personal qualities could help me meet life's challenges and attain my goals. So when I decided I should have a slimmer body like some of the girls I saw on television, I had no doubt I could "use my head" and in no time become just as thin. It was easy to find a diet and gain the approval of both myself and of others for doing the "right thing."

Unknowingly, this simple thought launched a ten-year struggle with my weight and my relationship to food. Even worse, as I gathered more information to fuel my thoughts of weight loss I completely dismissed the voice of my *best self*. Although I professed to have the same conviction as the Peanuts comic strip character Lucy screaming "I'm my own person" on a poster displayed at that time on my bedroom wall, my "own person" was nowhere to be found when it came to deciding what to eat. Diet rules not only determined what I ate, but also restricted how I lived each day of my life in my attempts to force myself to adhere to their rules. And there was never a shortage of diets to follow. When I failed to stick to one, there were always plenty more to choose from with new sets of instructions that promised even faster results.

Although I initially set out to lose five to ten pounds, my weight spanned a seventy-pound range as I tried one diet after another over the next ten years. I made forced choices about the foods I ate and followed unnatural eating plans, including liquid meals from a can. The harder I tried, the less I succeeded. No longer trusting my own abilities to make healthy and happy eating choices, I relied solely on the diet rules espoused by the latest experts to decide what to eat and evaluate what I had already eaten. Self-deprecating and obsessive thoughts about my failure to maintain weight loss multiplied and it soon consumed my life.

It was an accumulation of diet failures that finally led me to the realization that this way of thinking and living was not only creating an unhappy relationship with food, but also keeping me from enjoying my life. It was only when I began focusing my energy *away* from the goal of losing weight and *toward* choosing to eat as "my own person" again, that I reclaimed my natural relationship with food and experienced its ability to enhance the joy and meaning in my everyday life.

One by one, I let go of the life-restricting thoughts that had formed from eating with a focus on losing weight. I eliminated altogether my list of forbidden foods and all the rules that went with it. I ate for fun and for the taste of the food. I became involved in physical activities that I enjoyed and that integrated easily into my daily life. The seventy pounds I had struggled with for all those years vanished, along with my preoccupation with weight loss-focused eating. For the past thirty years, the eating experiences flowing from my *best self* have enriched my day-to-day life.

Delicious, fulfilling, scrumptious, mysterious, memorable, comforting, heart-warming, intuitive, pleasurable, nourishing, nurturing, and eye-opening are just a few words that describe the eating experiences that come about when food and our *best selves* naturally connect in the moment. Rather than being ruled by beliefs focused on the future promise of weight loss, our inner wisdom quietly talks to us through intuition, gut feelings, physical cravings, and thoughts based on our own experiences. It only follows that our best relationship with food emerges when we allow ourselves to consider all aspects of our lives that are present in the moment at hand as we are choosing to eat.

The purpose of this book is simply to remove these barriers that are preventing you from accessing and trusting your own inner wisdom as you choose and create each eating experience. A five-step guide provides the tools you need to remove the thoughts that are obstructing your inner wisdom and lead you back to everyday eating choices directed by your *best self*. Each chapter brings you one step closer to your natural relationship with food, that is, a connection that enhances your everyday life through deeper and more enjoyable eating experiences that are uniquely right for you.

Throughout the book, words are put together in phrases that emphasize a concept or make them easier to understand and remember; for example, the chapters form the acronym GUIDE, which stands for the following:

Goal-Replacing

Uncovering

Informing

Deciding

Experiencing

STEP I: Goal-Replacing Under the direction of your *best self,* allow your own natural relationship with food to emerge by no longer making food choices with the goal of losing weight.

STEP II: Uncovering Empty your mind of all weight loss-focused rules to discover your *best self.*

STEP III: Informing Provide your *best self* with information about you and your relationship with food that matters to you.

STEP IV: Deciding Make each eating decision under the direction of your *best self.*

STEP V: Experiencing Fully embrace all aspects of your life with food.

*Throughout this guide, you will find real life examples and tools on how to discover your own unique relationship with food. Watch for the following sections: Table, Self-Reflections, Personal Reflection, Take Action, Daily Reminder, and Self-Affirmations.

A Word of Encouragement

Accepting and embracing a new way of thinking about food and eating can be quite challenging. Enjoyable eating experiences may be followed by misdirected thoughts that pull you back into the world of rule-bound eating. Stay vigilant, but give yourself understanding when you find SAD beliefs attempting to regain their control over your relationship with food. Your *best self* will triumph and as its natural role in making eating choices strengthens, you will realize that none of your food desires need to be feared, but welcomed—they create enriching eating and living experiences. Keeping your *best self* in charge will enable you to choose the tools you want to use, not force you to follow established diet rules.

The discoveries may surprise you, not only will you experience a new relationship with food, but each eating experience will contribute to your new relationship with life.

AUTHOR'S NOTE

As you now turn the page to embark on your new journey with food, not only will the thoughts that you have about how to eat be challenged, but also you are likely to have expectations about how this book should be written. Perhaps you have already flipped to the back looking for recipes and discovered that they are not there. Or you may have skimmed the book expecting to find a sample weekly menu that isn't there either. And there are no charts to tell you the nutritional or caloric value or fat grams of the food that you eat. Are you hoping to find a page or two of particular foods that you "should and should not" eat, lists that are commonly found in the best-selling diet books? You won't find that in this book. As a matter of fact, you will see that there are absolutely no rules for you to follow in this book—with the possible exception of being instructed *not* to have any rules. What you will find at the end of the book, however, are self-affirmations that remind you that you already have all the answers you need and you do not need any of the things you might have been hoping or expecting to find in this book.

So as you turn each page, don't be surprised if you find yourself wanting more specific information. You may even believe that something throughout the entire book is missing. You are right, something is missing, but this lack of content is not a mistake or an oversight. The empty spaces that you find while reading this book are there for a reason: for you to complete. As this misdirected knowledge falls to the wayside, your inner wisdom is freed and has the chance to fill in the newly created spaces with eating experiences that are uniquely yours and enhance your everyday life. Only then can a natural relationship with food have a chance to emerge.

Finding your way back to *natural* means making choices that spring with ease from a place deep within you rather than from an artificial weight loss-focused construct. My hope is that you will welcome this unique reading experience, take the challenge and turn this book into your personal guide. My contribution to your journey is just a little more than a hundred pages. Your part, however, is full of unlimited possibilities that will not only improve your relationship with food, but enhance the quality of your everyday life, one eating experience at a time.

Quick Quiz:

What Kind of Eater Are You?

What does your current relationship with food look like? Are you a diet junkie? Take this quiz to discover what kind of eater you are. Keeping your quiz results in mind throughout the rest of this book may help you in determining how best to approach, think about, and resolve your struggling relationship with food.

Directions: *Answer* yes *or* no *to the following questions. On a separate sheet of paper, record your answers. For every question you answer* yes, *record a* 1. *If you answer* no, *record* 0. *At the end of the quiz, add your points together to obtain your* SAD Score. *Your total score will range from 0 to 30.*

1. Do you eat to lose weight?
2. Do you make eating choices based on fat and calorie content?
3. Do you spend time thinking about what you are going to eat, what you are not going to eat, or what you should not have eaten?
4. Do you choose certain physical activities over others in order to burn calories or fat?
5. Are you disturbed by the physical signs of weight fluctuation, such as bloating and tighter-fitting clothes?
6. Do you weigh yourself or monitor body fat on a regular or frequent basis?
7. Do you seem to spend most of your time trying to follow diet rules, breaking diet rules, or trying to maintain your weight?

8. When you are eating, do you make judgments about whether you are being good or bad?

9. Do you believe following diet rules is a natural part of a thin person's life?

10. Do you automatically order a diet soda, a salad with dressing on the side, or the low-fat or "skinny" platter when eating out?

11. Do you experience guilt if you eat solely based on pleasure or flavor, or if you eat when you are not particularly hungry?

12. Do you often hear yourself saying, "I should not have eaten that" about fattening foods?

13. Do you find yourself making plans around your eating rather than eating around your plans?

14. Do weight control thoughts and activities monopolize more of your time than you would like?

15. Do you try to make different arrangements if you feel your current plans may tempt you to break a diet rule?

16. Do you often engage in eating programs or diet plans with prescribed rules and guidelines?

17. Have you missed doing something you really wanted to do because you were afraid someone might notice that you gained weight?

18. Do you often plan the foods you will allow yourself to eat a day, a week, or even a month in advance?

19. Have you often found yourself referring to different times in your life in terms of the body size or weight that you were at that time?

20. Would you like diet rules to be a naturally integrated part of who you are?

21. Do you believe that there are people who will always have to watch their weight and you are one of them?

22. Do you feel you are letting yourself down if you make

an eating choice without considering its effect on weight loss?

23. Do you feel good about yourself when you decide to start a diet?

24. Do you believe that you will follow some diet rules for the rest of your life?

25. Do you ever call yourself a "food addict," a "compulsive eater," an "overeater," or a "diet failure"?

26. Do you consider sticking to a diet and losing weight a sign of character?

27. Do you believe that ideal dieting is eating only when you are hungry?

28. Do you believe that dieting to lose weight is a difficult but admirable thing to do?

29. Do you believe that people who are overweight should try to diet to lose weight?

30. Are there people in your life with whom you share weight loss experiences and diet stories?

Analyzing Your SAD Score

Your score shows to what degree you may knowingly or unknowingly be influenced by SAD in your everyday eating thoughts and behavior.

0 points = Best Self Eater. You have a natural relationship with food. You do not make eating choices with weight loss in mind. You listen to your inner wisdom and integrate the needs and desires from within, resulting in a harmonious relationship with food. You enjoy food. Your body size is most likely at its comfortable and natural weight.

1 to 10 points = Unsuspecting Influence.   Your eating choices are influenced by diet principles that you may not have realized you were maintaining. You may not consider yourself a dieter and probably do not engage in structured diet plans. Under this influence of SAD, your body size may not have found its natural and comfortable weight.

11 to 20 points = Under the Influence.   Food choices are a struggle for you. Artificial knowledge about dieting and weight loss is influencing living and eating choices that interfere with your ability to fully embrace what each day offers. Your current body size most likely does not reflect a natural weight for this time in your life.

21 to 30 points = Unnatural SAD Eater.   Conflicts and confusion about how, what, when, and where to eat are on your mind daily. You find yourself in continual food struggles that are unnatural and forced. SAD causes problems in other aspects of your life because the voice of your innermost wisdom is silenced. An erratic eating style (including anorexia nervosa and bulimia) may be present as unnatural eating interferes with your physical and emotional health. You are probably maintaining a significantly underweight or excessively overweight body. Or you may be constantly experiencing extreme weight fluctuations caused by weight loss-focused eating.

CHAPTER I

STEP 1: GOAL-REPLACING

The first step on the path to discovering your new life with food is to consider an entirely new purpose for eating; allow your own natural relationship with food to unfold, one eating experience at a time.

The Natural Way

So what do I mean by "natural?" I am not referring to the idea of avoiding foods with artificial flavors, processing, or added chemicals—that may or may not be a factor that affects your eating choices. A natural relationship with food consists of everyday eating experiences that are aligned with one's character or innate makeup, according to one's nature. Each of us already has the mechanism within us to make food choices that reflect who we are and the way we were meant to eat. So a natural relationship with food simply needs the chance to express itself; this happens when outcome-focused thoughts are stopped and all the factors that contribute to the moment at hand are considered when we eat. Rather than take control, judge, or condemn your desires to eat, your inner wisdom directs each eating experience. Your *best self* observes, accepts, and appreciates the role it plays in understanding the unique way that you were meant to eat.

You are likely to already have enjoyed natural eating experiences in your life. Like me, you may realize that you ate naturally up until your teenage years when you went on your first diet. Or maybe you have lived with only a few glimpses of what it is like to eat your own way and not according to rules or the direction of others. You may currently have a relationship with food that is centered on weight loss and until you picked up this book, you were not even aware of how unnatural it has become. Or perhaps, like me, you may find that most of the time your choices are coming from your inner wisdom but there is always more to discover that will continue to deepen the quality of this natural, life-enhancing relationship with food.

What would our relationship with food be like without the influence of today's society? Let's look back at our early food interactions and the workings of our own natural wisdom. Each person's relationship with food is unique within a natural process; each relationship is directed by our individual *best selves*. As infants, eating decisions are made primarily in response to physical instinct. When our stomachs are empty, it signals that it needs food, and we discover that we will get a response if we cry. We receive nourishment and our body and its natural processes indicate when we will stop eating. As we grow, other variables besides physical hunger contribute to our decisions about when and what we are going to eat. As children, we learn about textures and tastes, and we may connect certain foods with comfort and joy or with positive and negative events. We might eat too much candy and get a stomachache, or maybe we experiment with not eating enough in a given day and feel weak. Perhaps we want our favorite food every day or want to try a variety of unusual mixtures of tastes and textures. You may have shared lunch with a child trying new concoctions such as a potato chip dunked in root beer or a peanut butter and apple sandwich. Within the limits of the adult in charge, the eating possibilities of childhood are endless as we explore our foods.

During adolescence, our food choices often reflect emotional and social development. For example, adolescents may begin making their own lunches, choosing their own snacks in the cafeteria, or frequenting a popular fast-food restaurant with friends after school. During this time of life, it is easy to see how food choices add to and reflect our life experiences. Social and emotional associations with food become variables accessible to the *best self* as it makes its daily decisions. Adolescent eating styles may vary from three meals with the family one day to a day of junk food while shopping with friends at the mall.

The *best self* naturally has access to all of this information, not only considering our physical and emotional variables, but also our acquired ideas over the course of all our eating experiences. For example, we may receive a message from the stomach that the body is not completely satisfied and it craves a food with a sweet taste. We may see a television advertisement and be reminded of homemade cookies. We intuitively decide to eat a cookie without understanding all the ways it has enriched that particular life's moment. This can only occur when all information gathered by our *best self* (without the influences of restricting judgments and obstructing thoughts) and we are allowed to participate freely in each eating experience.

So are you ready to start where you left off, before thoughts based on weight loss were allowed to block your natural relationship with food? Contrary to what you might expect, one side effect of eliminating the goal of losing weight is the loss of diet-induced excess weight. As it becomes nutritiously fulfilled, the body can return to its natural metabolic rate and find its comfortable size. Guided by your inner wisdom, you may discover that your body size varies throughout different times of the year or with different life circumstances, or it may stay the same regardless of your varying eating experiences. The *best self* is aware that genetic influences, situational factors, life circumstances, and biological variations contribute to the way we eat and the way the body responds. We can get a better understanding of a natural relationship with food by looking at some other kinds of relationships that flow with ease under the direction of one's *best self,* such as the bond that is often shared with our animal companions that is exemplified in the following story:

> Alice has a loving and natural relationship with her cat that brings much joy to her life. With little thought or effort involved, she is responsive to his needs. Her love for animals, caring nature, and strong sense of responsibility all influence the daily choices that she makes. The cat responds and a changing natural relationship between the two of them emerges. Does she follow a specific structured program to ensure the proper development of the relationship? No. Alice has collected some information on cats and consults the veterinarian and other cat owners from time to time but she follows her own inclinations to love and care for her animal companion. Alice does not wake up every

morning confronting the issue of whether she is going to have enough willpower to stick to her plan of responsibility, nor does she plan how much time she is going to spend petting or talking to her cat. She allows the animal's mood and behavior, along with the other variables that enter her day, influence those decisions. Her experiences vary with each day as the activities in her life vary, and the relationship flows accordingly.

So what do Alice and her cat have to do with figuring out how to eat? With the new goal of discovering a natural relationship with food, you can expect a similar process to unfold. Everyday life consists of the flow of varying needs and desires of our body, mind, and soul—our deepest essence—as we interact with the world. When we ask ourselves the question "What eating experience do I want now?" we may naturally choose to address one need over another in that moment—no different than any choice made in our day. For example, when I choose to tend to my sick cat, my desire to play with my dog is put on hold. Likewise, when we drive a car we take a multitude of factors into account, often without even realizing the decision-making process that is happening within us. We consider the fact that there is a risk every time we get into a car. There are statistics about the chance of accidents under certain weather and road conditions. Sometimes, though, we may decide to drive on a dangerous street or try to get ahead of an upcoming storm to get to where we need to go. Allowing a natural relationship with food to unfold naturally is a similar process. Our particular eating choices on a given day vary depending on all of the other factors present in that moment. For example, the choice a *best self* might make during finals week at college may consist of many late nights of pizza with friends whereas the *best self* of an expectant mother may be to focus on the nutritional value of her food choices as she is considering not only her nutritional needs, but also those of her baby.

It all seems so simple and natural. So what happened? How did we lose this natural ability to make choices about eating? Throughout this century, society has promoted artificial and contrived goals for us when making food choices. An outlook on food that I have previously referred to as SAD, or Socially Acceptable Deprivation, has influenced those of us born in the twentieth century and onward. SAD requires us to make rule-bound eating choices for the purpose of losing weight. People commonly express dissatisfaction with their bodies and the desire to be thinner; going on a diet to lose weight is not an unusual decision and is still one of the most common New Year's resolutions. How many people do you know have tried to lose weight? Most people have been on at least one diet, and many individuals have made multiple attempts at following restrictive eating programs throughout their lifetime. Since there is nothing natural about eating to intentionally alter our bodies, we have had to turn to diet experts to tell us what to do, igniting the estimated fifty to sixty billion dollar a year diet industry.

Although there have been a number of anti-diet books published in the last decade, society continues to promote and support eating behavior based on weight loss. However, the general consensus of current research studies and surveys reveals that diets still do not work and it is commonly reported that even when there is a weight loss, it is regained within the year—ninety-five to ninety-eight percent of the time! Isn't it amazing how new weight loss programs still continue to spring up in spite of such an abysmal failure rate?

This outcome-focused way of thinking about food survives, and continues to thrive, in spite of its failure to achieve what it promises. Sadly, it feels more natural than ever to rely on external rules and restrictions than to listen to our own inner wisdom. Many individuals I have worked with have told me that giving up dieting feels strange. One twenty-year diet veteran told me that although she hated dieting, she liked the fact that it gave her the feeling that she was at least on the right track. It almost seems like a behavior that they love to hate, but continue to engage in with pride. Dieting to lose weight is so widely accepted as the norm that people are not even aware of the ways that it detracts from their experiences of food and of their everyday living.

So perhaps a look at the negative effects Socially Acceptable Deprivation, or SAD, has on our wellbeing can provide the impetus for re-thinking what we have been falsely led to believe is a healthy approach to eating. As soon as we focus on weight loss as our goal in eating, we set ourselves up to deprive the body, mislead the mind, and distract the soul, our innermost essence. SAD is hazardous to your health.

Studies throughout the last few decades have confirmed that restrictive eating causes the body to lower its metabolism and also triggers episodes of overeating. The body naturally responds to food deprivation as a threat to survival. It defends itself by decreasing the rate at which it burns calories in order to conserve energy, producing an unnatural state and slowing or altogether stopping any weight loss hoping to be achieved. For example, if you only have a cup of coffee and a piece of toast for breakfast and expect to get through a busy morning at work, your body will wisely conserve that fuel in order to continue functioning. In addition to a slowed metabolism, the body further responds to this unnatural state by sending out intense cravings for large amounts of food with high fat or high sugar contents, leading to diet-induced overeating. For example, if your semi-starved body has not been fed for several hours you are more likely to feel compelled to find fast food and quickly eat it in the car rather than taking the time to feel what your body really needs and then supplying it.

Besides leading us to falsely conclude that we will sustain a weight loss, dieting further encourages us to hold onto false ideas about ourselves in relation to our body size. "Quick fix" programs suggest that all kinds of wonderful things will be happening in our lives as soon as we reach that magic number on the scale. I interviewed college-aged women as part of my research for my doctoral dissertation. They commonly reported the belief that attaining their ideal weight would result in significant personality changes including feeling less hostile and depressed, as well as becoming more capable and independent. How many people do you know have expressed the thought that the social life that they have always dreamed of awaits them along with that perfect relationship as soon as they lose weight? Rather than questioning the validity of the promise of the better life through dieting, weight loss testimonials seem to only motivate dieters to never give up.

In addition to its false promises, dieting also deprives us of the simple and ordinary everyday pleasure of eating when we are hungry. By its very nature, dieting sets us up for an adversarial relationship with our hunger and our desire to eat good-tasting food. Sometimes a particular weight loss program even involves eating foods that we do not particularly like. Examples of such unpleasant eating experiences might include drinking powdered, tasteless diet drinks or a highly processed, artificially flavored, low-calorie and low-fat packaged meal made with absolutely no regard to the eater's interests and preferences. Since the goal is to lose weight at all costs, many dieters start to believe that it is always a good idea to try to eat as little as possible or not at all. With this construct in mind, the feelings of hunger are not only unwelcomed, but they create anxiety. Hunger cues and cravings are no longer appreciated as part of the natural workings of the body telling you to stop what you are doing and take in the pleasures of an eating experience. A desire for a food item that is not part of the plan you are following automatically falls under the category of something to be fought or ignored. But the detrimental effects on your sense of self do not stop with the daily struggles and tension around eating. Since resisting the natural inclinations to eat satisfying, fulfilling, and enjoyable food feels like the right thing to do, remorse and disappointment are likely to set in when you lose one of these battles. Should we ask a psychologist if such daily conflict around such a natural everyday part of being alive can possibly be good for one's mental health and sense of self?

Not only does weight loss-focused eating detract from the simple enjoyment of eating, it blocks the chance for the soul—our deepest essence where intuitive wisdom lies—to naturally express itself in our food choices. Since we have already seen how our whole person—body, mind, and soul—contributes to and enhances our eating experiences, it only follows that the choices we make about food hold valuable information about our unique innermost being. But we block the receiving of that unique insight by stopping the fulfilling of those desires when they arise with a dieting rule. Likewise, we shut down the attempts our soul may have to express its uniqueness through our food choices that may not conform to the latest diet we are following. For example, instead of considering that our craving for chocolate might be a desire to sweeten a harsh and bitter day, we ignore the urge altogether because we have forbidden ourselves to eat this delicacy because of the amount of fat or calories it contains. The mysterious language of the soul expressed through food cravings gets lost as rules shutting down the vast possibilities of self-understanding that is being offered to us.

Personal Reflection

The following personal story illustrates how weight loss-focused eating can distract the soul from its ability to create and enjoy our life's experiences. I was just ending an "egg-grapefruit" diet when my sister told me she was getting married in six months and wanted me to be her maid of honor. My first thought was that I needed to restrict my eating even more severely in order to lose weight more quickly. I lost twenty pounds in two months. Four months later, my sister's wedding date arrived; however, I had regained not only all the weight I had lost, but an additional fifteen pounds as well. At the time, I thought this was a devastating tragedy, but I realize now that the real misfortune was that I missed the full experience of my sister's wedding and the days leading up to it by spending all my time concentrating on losing weight or lamenting my weight gain instead of focusing on the celebration. Has dieting kept you from taking in the richness of life's special moments? Would you like to take this fullness of life back into your life?

Self-Reflections

Now that you have removed the goal of weight loss from your thoughts, ask yourself "What eating experience do I want now?" Consider the following aspects of a natural relationship with food and how they might influence eating experiences that consider the needs and desires of your whole person—the body, mind, and soul. While finding your natural relationship with food is likely to change your body size, keep the goal of weight loss off your list of factors to consider when allowing your *best self* to make food choices.

For the body:

- Enjoy good health, longevity, and comfort
- Explore nonfood-related ways to have a healthy body
- Enjoy good health and comfort
- Reduce health risk factors that run in the family
- Increase fruits, vegetables, grains, and fiber for better functioning
- Experiment with ways to nourish the body with nutrients, minerals and vitamins

For the mind:

- Think clearly and have energy

• Be realistic about goals for being "healthy"
• Explore what to do with the time, energy, and money no longer spent on dieting
• Take the time to explore the adventure of different foods
• Explore personal freedom of choice

For the soul:

• Allow food to add pleasure to everyday life
• Be at peace with food and enjoy eating
• Have a better understanding of self, others, and the world
• Accept the mystery of some food experiences

TAKE ACTION

1. Take some time to consider and write down some of your new desires for your unique relationship with food. What does the list look like? These are your new desires, not your goals. They do *not* need to be achieved by certain dates to be considered a success. These desires are in a constant state of change.

2. Put away the scale and the weight charts and any other items you have that measure your steps toward the goal of weight loss.

3. Identify ways that SAD eating may have caused you to miss out on the complete experience of a significant life event. Had you realized it at the time? Was it worth it?

4. Ask yourself "What eating experience do I want now?" every time you eat.

DAILY REMINDER

I am not making food choices to lose weight. I am discovering new experiences with food every day.

CHAPTER II

STEP 2: UNCOVERING

Discover the Voice of Your *Best Self*

At this point, you might be asking, "What is this *best self* that I am looking for and how do I know when I find it?"

You are rediscovering your inner wisdom, that is, your *best self*, a concept that has existed since ancient times. Over the years, it has been referred to in a variety of ways, including your highest self, essence, the nameless, being, true nature, depth, an intuitive knowing, divine spirit within, and the soul. Regardless of what we choose to call it, this universal teaching espouses that our natural inclination is to fully embrace all that life offers, one moment at a time. This creates a natural flow of experiences. This innate ability to respond to life does not require studying with a spiritual teacher or reading certain books; it is already within each of us. It becomes blocked, however, by the engrained and artificial thought systems that we have come to rely upon that focus our attention on the past or on attaining a future outcome rather than taking in what is present. It is only in letting go of these obstructing thoughts that we can once again hear the unique voice within each of us that creates interactions with the world that are aligned with our true nature.

Expanding upon these ideas, I have identified three guiding forces that are present when our *best self*, as I see it, is directing our everyday life experiences, including eating. For simplicity in understanding, I call them "The Three As": Authenticity, Acceptance, and Appreciation.

1. Authenticity

Experiencing life with authenticity calls us to recognize who we truly are, including traits that we are pleased with and others we might not find so desirable. It is about letting you freely be all that you are. Your *best self* chooses to acknowledge and accept all of you—your needs, wants, and vulnerabilities. It is not being afraid to see what is real even when it may present a conflict in one's view of a current situation. For example, a naturally creative person may experience frustration in a job requiring routine and precision. Perhaps the position offers her the security she desires, but recognizing how it is holding her back from her natural form of expression might cause her to seriously consider a career change. Or, let's look at the grandmother whose daughter believes that if she was any kind of loving and caring person, she should enjoy babysitting her grandchildren on a regular basis. But this grandmother does not find it to be naturally pleasurable. So rather than denying her feelings, this grandmother's courage to accept them in spite of her daughter's views, will allow her to best consider all options when finding a compromise that works for everyone. Furthermore, it is only when we acknowledge and accept an aspect of ourselves that we find to be limiting that we give ourselves the chance to find the gift that may also be present within this initially unwelcomed discovery of our true self. For example, an individual whose learning style required him to work harder as a child to succeed, may find that because of his challenge he developed the perseverance that helped him attain the career he wanted as an adult.

So how can an eating choice detract from honoring our true self? Dieting can keep us from embracing our authenticity; the extent to which this happens varies depending on the influence SAD has had in our lives. Without even realizing it, the focus on the outcome of weight loss can cause us to lose sight of the true nature of who we are. For example, a person who loves to dance may no longer recognize her fondness for this kind of self-expression because she has become self-conscious about her body size. The thoughts created from her failed dieting efforts win. Dieting also allows us to put off facing traits in ourselves that we do not particularly like because we expect them to go away when we lose the excess weight.

Self-Reflections

Consider becoming reacquainted with your authentic self by asking yourself the following questions without allowing any of the weight loss-focused thoughts contributing to the answers: What do you value most in your life? What matters to you? What are your unique and perhaps eccentric traits? When do you feel most yourself?

What drives you crazy about you? In what way could you courageously show others who you really are?

2. Acceptance

Living with acceptance means taking in all that life offers without resistance, even those experiences that we label as bad. While we do not have to like it or even condone it, the *best self* chooses to accept, without resistance, what *is*. It can be a challenging task as life often brings us what we did not want, from a friend's betrayal, a job layoff, or a failed relationship, to floods and tornados, war, or an unexpected illness or accident. When we accept what is, we stop the complaining, the "what if" sentiments, and the regretful stream of thought often laced with tremendous amounts of fear and trepidation as to what will happen next. When the *best self* is in charge, that obstructing negativity is replaced with a willingness to accept our feelings about the situation and then make our best response given whatever it is that happened.

How does SAD eating interfere with acceptance? When we are dieting, we hold on to the false promises of weight loss, the impression that "things will be better than they are now when I lose weight" and so we are able to put off the disenchantment of reality. We do not face what is real because we grasp onto a sense of false control over life's happenings. We are distracted from what the present event is asking us to see because we stay focused on the future and our fantasy that we can control by getting stricter on our diets and losing weight.

Self-Reflections

Practice acceptance in your life by asking yourself the following questions without allowing your SAD beliefs about yourself contribute to the answers: What drives you crazy about people and the world? What kinds of things happened unexpectedly in your life? Are you aware of an area in your life that you are choosing not to see it for what it really is? Where has life disappointed you? Where has life pleasantly surprised you?

3. Appreciation

Experiencing life with appreciation means welcoming the complexities of the human experience as life unfolds. Life happens. And just like the challenge of acceptance, living with appreciation means staying open to the gifts of life even when things are not happening as we expected, hoped for, or possibly even worked very hard to attain. Perhaps what you thought were your personal needs and desires may seem to find no fulfillment in your current life conditions. Or you may feel blindsided when you realize that even though you gave all you had to a relationship that you approached with your generous, compromising, and loving nature it seemed to bring you only sadness and despair. Years later, however, in the spirit of appreciation you realize how not getting what you thought you so desperately wanted brought your life to a much more rewarding place than you ever could have imagined. You may see what you perceived as an obstacle turn into the stepping stone of a dream right before your eyes. For example, an individual may reluctantly accept a job transfer to a new city they had not considered living in, but later find their future partner in that location and fulfill their vision for a family. Your inner wisdom is also able to appreciate the growth in personal strength and the development of the ability to compromise or improvise in the face of adversity. We may not welcome the painful challenges that being human can bring, but deep within we know that there are positive elements that can be found or can come out of even our darkest times. Living with appreciation means realizing that sometimes we are faced with situations that have no easy answers, quick fixes, or resolutions that we find acceptable. In other words, appreciation gives us the chance to find both the pain and the gift in a challenging situation.

What role does appreciation have in our eating experiences? Once again, living with SAD blocks our ability to appreciate life's moments and our responses to them. The focus on dieting obscures our recognition of a situation's complexity as the ingrained diet beliefs narrow our range of emotional responses to it. We are happy and proud of ourselves when we get on the scale and see a weight loss and we are disappointed in ourselves and adjust our plans accordingly when our weight is higher than it was the last time. We may even have that number on the scale determine what decisions we make about what else we are doing later that day. SAD determines the range of our emotional responses to life. The insistence that by controlling what we eat and what we weigh will get us what we want leaves no room for growing as a person, finding gifts in challenging situations, or learning to go with the flow.

Self-Reflections

To reconnect with your inner wisdom's sense of appreciation, think back on a time in your life where disappointment and loss opened the door for new adventure and joys. Can you identify personal strengths that surfaced from a difficult struggle? Can you identify the "blessings in disguise" in your life?

Giving Up the Obstructing Way

Emptying your mind of all the rules of weight loss-focused eating uncovers the *best self*'s ability to apply these three guiding forces to your relationship with food. When your energy is harnessed into a diet-compelled lifestyle your ability to fully experience the uniqueness in yourself, your life, and the greater human experience is highly limited. Remove from your mind all the knowledge that obstructs the natural way and put your *best self* in charge. To begin uncovering, we need to identify and understand our misconceptions about eating and ourselves that impede our natural relationship with food.

While we are all influenced by a society that promotes eating based on weight loss, that is Socially Acceptable Deprivation (SAD), the impact of this misdirected thinking on our relationship with food varies from individual to individual. Some people have lives engulfed by prescribed diets and sacred eating rules, while others are rule-bound eaters who do not label themselves as dieters but regularly restrict their food choices to "watch" their weight. Many ex-dieters limit their eating experiences by unknowingly continuing to follow rules and restrictions ingrained in their minds. Others say they have given up on losing weight; they do not diet and they do not lose weight. This self-defeating mindset taints their eating experiences with guilt, feelings of failure and dislike or even hatred for their bodies. Weight loss-focused eaters may have body sizes ranging from life-threateningly underweight to significantly and medically overweight. There are individuals of all sizes who eat without giving much thought to the value and pleasure of food in their lives. Although eating styles and body sizes vary, all of these eaters are experiencing interference in their natural relationship with food.

In spite of the variance to which people are influenced by SAD, I have found there to be three common characteristics that are always present and made up of obstructing thoughts and behaviors: social identity, obsession, and loss of freedom. Each of these ways of approaching food choices not only blocks access to your inner wisdom, but also diminishes the quality of everyday life experiences by interfering with your *best self*'s access to its life-guiding forces, "The Three As": Authenticity, Acceptance, and Appreciation. Each of the three obstacles is maintained by an underlying false belief promoted by modern society that corresponds with one of the "The Three As." Understanding the misdirected thinking that maintains each obstacle will allow you to remove them and let go of SAD. As you read the following descriptions, notice which thoughts and behaviors you recognize in yourself.

The Three Obstacles

1. **Social Identity**
2. **Obsession**
3. **Loss of Freedom**

OBSTACLE 1: Social Identity

What it looks like: You identify yourself as a dieter. Your goals in losing weight impact your self-image. Your eating decisions begin with the thought "I should . . ." You assume that striving to make food decisions for weight control will always be a factor in how you perccive yourself. You accept the widely available and socially supported belief that dieting is a positive lifestyle rather than recognizing it as a problem and an obstruction to your authentic self. You find social reinforcements for dieting even when it is not working. When you regain weight, you look to the diet community for support and find a new program that promises to work.

When thinking about your life, you associate different events with your body weight or diet status. You can identify the diets you have been on, fluctuations in your weight, and the events in your life at each weight:

I was a size five for Homecoming, but a size nine for the prom.

I met John while I was on the Beverly Hills diet, and I fell in love with Bob after I finished a seven-day

45

liquid diet.

The Thanksgiving to Christmas stretch was just a nightmare and I couldn't even zip up the dress I had worn the previous New Year's Eve.

I remember getting on the scale at the health club the day that I applied for that new job. I weighed 127.5 pounds.

You do not feel complete unless you are following diet rules. Dieting is a significant part of your self-concept, and you experience symptoms of withdrawal when separated from its belief system.

The underlying false belief for individuals who identify themselves as dieters is that it is *desirable* for SAD to be a natural part of their everyday life. They are proud to be identified by their eating decisions that aim to control their weight. They turn to following rules for their sense of self. In reality, however, this externally imposed identity distracts them from uncovering their authenticity.

How Social Identity Blocks Authenticity

When you are caught up in the social identity of a SAD lifestyle your true self is suppressed. Rather than coming to terms with those traits that are more challenging to accept, you can falsely hold onto the belief that you will be different once you lose weight. While you wait for your body to transform, you hold onto a false sense of self by blaming your negative traits on body size. When you believe losing weight will remove your "bad" qualities you never have to face them or integrate them into your true self. The following examples illustrate how we can inadvertently block the deeper aspects of our authentic selves by hiding behind the superficial identity of a dieter. In all of the following cases, these individuals chose to avoid the anxiety that may often come along with discovering the more challenging aspects of one's true nature. Rather than taking this discomfort as an opportunity to find a deeper understanding of themselves, they blocked further self-exploration by choosing to resolve any conflicts that they felt with the decision to simply become a better dieter.

> Kevin was afraid to commit himself to a relationship with a woman he was dating. He decided to wait until he lost weight and was in excellent physical shape before considering a stronger commitment to the relationship. With this decision, Kevin was able to use his beliefs about dieting to avoid the challenge of becoming more vulnerable, thus blocking his *best self*'s desires for a closer relationship and all that it could bring to his life.

> Martha strongly identified with being a dieter. She described feeling "a sense of relief" each Sunday night after she planned the diet that would start the following Monday morning. She would allow herself one last night of "undisciplined eating," feeling reassured that she was still a dieter.

> Sarah, a participant in one of my workshops, reported feeling "great despair" when she first decided to quit dieting. She did not know what to eat or when to eat, and was at a loss as to what she should do now that she was no longer dieting. She didn't know if she could trust

herself to make the right decisions. Who was she if she was not a dieter? She then identified herself as a failure because she had given up on dieting. Her first inclination to fight this anxiety was to go back on a diet. She turned back to rules about eating after only a few attempts to give them up. Although she knew that her old lifestyle only presented more problems, she needed her immediate diet "fix" to relieve her anxiety.

OBSTACLE 2: Obsession

What it looks like: Your feelings, thoughts, and behaviors related to changing your weight have become obsessive. Weight control is the main consideration when you decide what and when to eat. You consume food that is not nutritiously adequate but temporarily fools your body into feeling full. You ingest common "filler" foods such as diet drinks, low-calorie gelatin, artificially sweetened candy, rice cakes, and a variety of nonfat, chemically altered items. Modern technology makes it easier to maintain this detailed obsession. You can buy an app for your phone that allows you to enter a food item you might be considering eating and get an entire page of facts about it. There are programs that add and subtract calories for you and basically tell you what to eat or not to eat next. Plug in some numbers on your computer and through some magic formula you will know exactly what you need to do to reach exactly what weight by exactly what date.

Exercise may become as much of a preoccupation as the food you eat. Modern exercise machinery tells you exactly how many calories you have burned while rowing, running, or walking on a treadmill. It is popular these days to wear a small device that measures your activity for you and translates the information into a suggestion about how many calories were burned while doing that activity. Enjoyment in the activity is not a priority.

The underlying false belief for individuals motivated by obsession is that all eating decisions should be based on weight control and body size alteration.

How Obsession Blocks Acceptance

Obsession in SAD masks your ability to accept life events through constant, repetitive diet beliefs and unbending goals surrounding weight loss in regards to dieting. Holding on to the idea that things will be better when you lose weight may replace your acceptance of a reality that is difficult to face. Diet rules are sometimes able to distract you from the pain of recognizing shattered hopes and dreams. You may choose to believe that things will work out if you follow your diet regimen and lose weight. For example, you go on a diet if you find yourself in a dissatisfying relationship. Rather than looking at other courses of action, you may choose to believe that your interpersonal problems will resolve themselves when you lose weight. Until those pounds are lost, you do not have to feel the letdown of a relationship that just did not work out. The *best self*'s desire for acceptance is never realized. The following stories exemplify the way in which people rely on diets to avoid dealing with conflicts and obstacles in their lives, never allowing their *best self* to face the challenge of acceptance.

Maria went to Hollywood when she was eighteen,

planning to find her ideal job: acting. When she was not immediately discovered as an actress she decided it was because she needed to lose weight. She came to believe that when she lost enough weight, and thus improved her body image, she would get her big movie break and become famous. Maria eventually returned to her hometown and seven years later she was still trying to lose weight. She continued to talk about her desire to return to Hollywood, further influencing her dieting decisions and rekindling her drive to lose weight and become an actress. Because Maria's obsession to lose weight was her only motivation behind procuring her dream job, she did not find other ways to become an actress. Her obsession ultimately prevented her from going after what she wanted in life rather than accepting herself and pursuing other means of following her dreams or listening to her *best self* to reassure her of her dreams of becoming a Hollywood actress.

Martha decided that she needed to make dieting a priority because she believed her boyfriend would love her more if she weighed less. Holding on to the false hope that she had found the perfect relationship, and that she wanted to foster it by any means necessary, was easier than facing and coming to terms with the fact that her relationship was failing because of reasons other than her weight.

Sandy was fourteen when she began to diet obsessively. Her parents were contemplating divorce, and it was too painful for Sandy to accept the adversity of her family's splitting apart. She thought that her parents might stay together if she could become thin. Her parents' inevitable divorce was clearly out of her control; however, excessive dieting allowed her to become distracted from her feelings about the divorce, exercise her own control of the situation through the rules of a diet, and to hold onto the idea that she could prevent it, rather than understand and accept the divorce.

After discovering she did not make the gymnastics team, Donna believed it was because of her weight. Determined to lose weight, she set unrealistic goals for herself that would allow her to become a champion gymnast. Soon, Donna became unnaturally obsessive about her relationship with food. She kept extensive diet records and thought she could trace any fluctuation in weight to a particular snack or meal. Her list of forbidden foods included items that tasted delicious to her but did not give her the feeling of being full. Donna became driven to learn the details about the content of food and began measuring exact portions. She recalled crying after realizing she mistakenly drank a bottle of non-diet soda. Obsessive dieting only postponed her need to perhaps adjust her dream of becoming a champion gymnast. This unhealthy obsession prevented her from seeing the reality of her situation and delayed her exploration of enjoying and excelling in other sports. She never made it to the Olympics, but as she let go of the dieting, she discovered her interest and natural talent for acting and enjoyed performing in her high school's plays.

OBSTACLE 3: Loss of Freedom

What it looks like: Dieting thoughts and behavior are part of your daily patterns. You are usually on a diet, breaking one diet and moving on to the next, or trying either to maintain a certain weight from a previous diet or to prevent weight gain following a "failed" diet. Scanning nutrition labels for grams of fat, carbohydrates, sugar, and other elements is automatic. You routinely categorize food choices as good or bad. Drinking excessive amounts of diet soda and coffee or chewing gum are automatic decisions you make in a constant attempt to sublimate your unwanted urges to eat. When you go out to eat severely limiting your choices is second nature. Instead of ordering something you know you will really enjoy, you make a decision based on what you think you should eat as dictated by your current diet plan, ordering the light or low-calorie platters or salads with dressing on the side. You may not go out at all so as to maintain control over your diet, declining invitations from friends to eat out or to go to a barbeque with family in order to prevent yourself from being subject to the temptation of eating foods you think you shouldn't. Your perceived progress—or lack of progress—on a diet may influence which social events you attend. You may cancel plans to go on a vacation to a warm climate where more revealing clothes are worn.

You have given up the freedom to choose based on hunger, taste, spontaneity, emotion, or situation. Your diet thoughts, analysis, and judgments diminish your freedom to also choose other ways to spend your time. These soul-stripping habits go beyond your food choices: you judge yourself by your eating behavior.

Dieting may significantly narrow the way you live. I have seen one's view of their weight affect their decision to apply for a job, go to the doctor, speak at a friend's wedding, or even visit a dying relative. You have given up freedom of choice in your eating and in your living.

The underlying false belief for people living with

the loss of freedom induced by dieting is that it is *desirable* to have a predetermined eating plan for weight control, and the more rigid the plan the better. As people surrender their freedom to SAD, they place their trust in external authority rather than inner wisdom. They allow their eating plans to affect other life decisions, limiting the possibilities that life offers.

How Loss of Freedom Blocks Appreciation

When we give up our freedom to SAD we limit the different ways we can explore a situation's complexities and mysteries. Dieting beliefs and its associated behaviors attempt to simplify the complexities of eating while progressing toward an end goal. However, these actions also narrow the range of our living experiences. Turning to eating rules rather than listening to your inner voice may help us avoid difficult decisions in the short term, but at the cost of silencing the true desires of the body and the soul. Dieting closes us off from accessing our *best selves*.

When we are under the influence of false diet beliefs we restrict our range of emotional and physical reactions, blocking our natural ability to fully experience life. We avoid the wide array of enriching experiences that life offers by limiting our freedom to choose as we wish. By focusing on only controlling our body size, we limit our ability to address and appreciate all that is present in that moment.

We know what to expect when following SAD: we are proud when we step on the scale and see that we have lost weight, and we are disappointed when we see the numbers on the scale rise. Determination to start over on a diet or to try a new one is not new to us, and there are few, if any, surprises left. Dieting allows us to forego the intensity of our natural responses and avoid unknown emotional and physical reactions. As illustrated in the following examples, this limited range of experience may give us a false sense of control over our feelings, but we have merely lost touch with the depths of our souls.

> One of my clients, a ten-year-old girl, was dealing with some difficult issues regarding her relationship with her mother, stepmother, father, siblings, and stepsiblings. One day she came into the session proudly announcing that she was on a diet because she wanted to lose weight. Since she was obviously a slender girl, I questioned her about her decision. She replied, "It's not that I'm fat. It is a healthy thing to do and will help me deal with my problems better." At age ten, she was already using dieting to provide a false sense of control over her problems.

> Influenced by SAD, my client Molly gave up her freedom to arrive at work on time and her choice to socialize with her coworkers. Molly was late for work on Wednesdays because it was an office tradition for her manager to bring pastries and doughnuts for everyone. Molly's dieting rules never allowed her to have pastries, or any food before noon for that matter. She believed, as influenced by her diet, that waiting as long as she could before beginning to eat every day was the fastest way to lose weight. Molly was ignoring her body's physical needs for sustenance in the morning, so with a body lacking fuel for energy, it is not surprising that she found it hard to resist the treats when they passed by her desk. Rather than having to squelch her desire to eat or contemplating ways to justify eating a doughnut or pastry, she was deliberately late for work on Wednesdays to avoid the temptation altogether.

Comparison of SAD with *Best Self* Eating

SAD	*BEST SELF*
listens to external authority	listens to inner authority
makes general rules for all	considers unique needs and desires
minds are filled with diet knowledge	minds are emptied of misleading diet information
deprived body	energized body
deceived mind	enlightened mind
distracted soul	enjoyment for the soul
rigidity in eating	flexibility in eating
encourages feelings of guilt and shame, false control, and failure	encourages the authentic self, acceptance of life, and appreciation of life's complexities
time-limited plans	everyday eating experiences
unnatural eating that masks feelings	natural eating that enhances feelings
harnesses energy into eating concerns	frees energy to explore authentic concerns
adversarial relationship with food	peaceful relationship with food
focuses on outcome: weight loss	trusts and enjoys the process of body, mind, and soul working together
unnatural excess weight	natural loss of unnatural diet-induced weight and unnatural diet-induced weight ideals

TAKE ACTION:
Five Techniques for Undoing SAD Thinking

Remove the misguided thoughts that obstruct the natural way. You have already started this journey by identifying the obstacles that interfere with your natural eating. Realizing that you may need to give up everything you have believed about how and what to eat may feel like a daunting task. But that awareness alone will give your natural relationship the freedom to come forth. Be gentle and patient with yourself through this process. Think of the following five techniques as a jumpstart to your new and natural approach to eating. Choose the ideas that will help you take action to free your *best self* from the misguided thoughts of SAD.

1. Remove the **Social Identity** obstacle and embrace **Authenticity**. Commit to finding your true desires in each eating experience.

To reverse the obstacle of identifying yourself as a dieter, you need to not consider weight control as a factor in your eating choices. Each choice is part of your unfolding relationship with food. Start by avoiding situations that highlight your identity as a person who monitors both the weight-related qualities of food (e.g., calories) and the bodily signs of weight loss (e.g., inches). Avoid any situation that tempts you to judge your food intake in any way at all. Avoid diet books and other paraphernalia designed to help you lose weight. Avoid exercise programs and motivational speakers that claim they can increase your willpower to diet. Avoid diehard dieters, or at least conversations with them about eating. Avoid the diet food aisle in the grocery store. Avoid any diet clubs or diet support groups you have joined. Avoid the restaurants that you frequented while dieting, or at least avoid ordering the diet meals. Increase the time you spend in non-diet-related activities that you enjoy.

Avoid any situation that tempts you to measure your body or focus attention on altering your body through weight control. Avoid the doctor's scale, the health club scale, your home scale, or the one at your friend's house. Avoid weight charts, tape measures, and skin calipers. Avoid wearing any clothes that feel too tight. Keep your immediate wardrobe stocked with comfortable clothes that fit. Spend less time in front of the mirror. Avoid exercise groups and people who talk about how much weight they have gained or lost and where it shows on their bodies. Avoid people who identify you as a dieter.

Perhaps you are thinking that all this avoidance will drastically change your present, familiar way of life. The point is to give up the artificial ways of identifying and judging yourself so your natural experiences with food have a chance to emerge. When you feel strong enough to embrace your new approach to eating, you will encounter these situations confidently. For example, you can make a *best self* choice about having dessert with friends. What a great way to announce your rejection of diet-focused thoughts! The action that my client Lisa took at work is a wonderful example of the effectiveness of this technique:

> Lisa, a high school teacher, considered the ability to diet a positive aspect and counted it as one of her strengths. When she let go of her dieter's status, she discovered her previously unhealthy identity was being reinforced in the teacher's lounge. She noticed that

most teachers were unnatural eaters and praised each other for the low-fat and low-calorie choices they made, which usually included some combination of the following: low-fat yogurt, sandwiches on thinly sliced bread, low-fat bagels, apples, rice cakes, and carrot sticks. At first, Lisa felt her coworkers would think she had given up on herself if they saw that she was no longer engaging in diet behavior. So she chose to have lunch and take breaks in her classroom until she felt strong enough to withstand the peer pressure to diet. When she chose to rejoin them later, she was able to enjoy her varying eating choices while accepting her coworkers place on their journey with food.

Self-Reflections

Questions to consider:

How has dieting become part of who you are?

In what situations do you label yourself as a dieter or a weight watcher?

Do you hide eating behavior that does not fit with your identity as a dieter?

How much does your success at dieting determine how you feel about yourself?

What would it be like to remove dieting from your identity?

DAILY REMINDER:

I will proudly display my identity as a non-dieter. I will let others know I am no longer willing to settle for the life of a dieter.

2. Counter the **Obsession** obstacle and return to **Acceptance**. Taste the forbidden.

This technique may surprise you. The elimination of obsession starts with the recognition that no foods are forbidden. Of course, this technique may require necessary restrictions when there are certain medical conditions such as diabetes or food allergies involved. Deciding to not eat certain foods for medical reasons is a constraint honored by the *best self*. This is a choice you are making for the betterment of your health, not a rule restricting your freedom of choice. A food is not to be forbidden, however, because of concerns about gaining weight. No particular food in and of itself, will cause you to gain weight. No certain place where you eat makes you gain weight. No particular time of day that you eat results in weight gain.

Start by eliminating the list of "rules that forbid." There can no longer be forbidden foods, places, or times to eat. Food choices can no longer be right or wrong. You may drink regular soda. Put sugar on your cereal. Butter your toast. Put real cream in your coffee. Have dressing and croutons on your salad. Eat a piece of candy. Enjoy a piece of birthday cake. Order French fries with your sandwich, which might even have mayonnaise on it. Have brownies, cupcakes, and cookies. You are now free to consider any of these as options. You may also eat any time of the day or night. You may eat after nine o'clock in the evening. You may even get up in the middle of the night and eat. Go ahead and eat five minutes after you have already eaten or eat before you go out to dinner. You may eat right before you are going to put on a tight dress. You may eat before a dance. You may eat before a doctor's appointment. Have dessert first if you wish. Have a second dessert immediately following the first dessert. You may eat first thing in the morning although you have eaten late the night before. You may eat after you have had second helpings. Go ahead and eat after you have put the food away. You may eat a fattening food on the first day of January. You may eat desserts on the first of the month, the first of the week, or on a Monday that happens to fall on the first day of the month (a tempting time to start one of those thirty-day diets). To really let yourself know that you are committed to tasting the forbidden, these are particularly good times to exercise your freedom to eat freely.

It is also important to eliminate forbidden *places* to eat. This means you may eat in your car. You may eat in the store, and you may even go grocery shopping when you are hungry. You may go to the drive-thru window of a fast-food restaurant and eat in the parking lot. You may eat while you are reading. You may eat while you watch television or when you are doing homework. You may eat at the kitchen table or on the living room couch. Go ahead and eat while you cook or while you clear the table. Eat while browsing the refrigerator.

Does this technique sound sacrilegious to you? You may discover that you rarely, if ever, even want to make any of the choices discussed above, especially some of the ides that may seem extreme to you—and that is fine. The point is that you can now eat any way that you want to. No eating option is forbidden by you or anyone else.

Removing all artificial restrictions is necessary before your *best self* can take charge of your natural relationship with food. The following story about a woman named Jane illustrates how her focus on forbidden foods inadvertently caused overeating:

> Jane's list consisted of treats she regularly craved that she believed triggered her to binge. Jane realized that after eating one of these items she often ate large amounts of other foods from her list that she did not even want. Sometimes she would eat any food that happened to be around. Because she became angry with herself for bingeing, she did not feel satisfied after eating that particular food. Guilt, shame, and often an upset stomach were her only rewards. Jane began her new adventure in eating by removing chocolate chip cookies and non-diet sodas from her list of forbidden foods. She was surprised how quickly the natural eating process began when she allowed herself to eat chocolate chip cookies and have regular soft drinks. When she finally allowed herself to have as many cookies as she wanted, she always ate fewer than she had anticipated. The first time she allowed herself to eat cookies, it seemed she wanted ten, so she ate ten. To her surprise, she felt uncomfortably full. She realized that she did not really want that many, but was testing her newly found freedom. When she set no limits, she quickly learned to listen to her body signal the number of cookies that would satisfy her craving. Jane also realized that when she drank the soda that contained sugar her sweet tooth was satisfied and she usually ate less food with her soft drink. Her craving for soft drinks completely diminished when she realized that usually her urge for diet soda was really a hunger signal. Dieting had caused her to try to fill normal hunger pangs with abnormal amounts of diet drinks. Jane

discovered that when she removed a food she often craved from the forbidden list it only took small amounts to satisfy her cravings for them.

Self-Reflections

Questions to consider:

What forbidden foods are on your current list?

Are there places you forbid yourself to eat?

Are there times you forbid yourself to eat?

DAILY REMINDER:

My body has been deprived of the pleasure of eating this forbidden food without guilt. My body needs time to accept that I am going to allow it to have this food. I will give myself some time to adjust to this new freedom so I can discover how this food will become part of my natural eating style.

3. Reverse the **Loss of Freedom** obstacle and return to **Appreciation**. Have learning days, not bad days.

Dieters describe the times that they deviate from their pre-scribed diets as "bad days." This third technique is designed to break the habit of automatically evaluating a food's calorie and fat content. Instead of judging yourself, learn from yourself. During your transition period from unnatural to *best self* eating, your food experiences will provide valuable information about your physical and emotional responses to what you consume. You can observe the natural rhythms of your body and learn how it works when it is hungry and when it is full. You may discover that some foods fill you up more quickly than others. You may determine which foods are difficult for your system to digest. You may find that you are a person who likes to have something sweet every day. You may realize that you feel better when you eat a meal in the morning, or learn that you sleep better on a full stomach. You may learn that some foods you used to crave are now too rich. You may also find out that once your body is convinced it is not going to be punished with starvation when it eats something sweet, it takes a smaller amount of sugar to satisfy your craving.

These new learning days may also teach you about your emotions. You may learn that when you are nervous you crave "finger food," or maybe you do not feel hungry at all. Perhaps you will find that you eat to relieve boredom. You may realize that you eat until you feel sick when you are trying to suppress angry feelings or have done something that goes against your values. You may learn that you eat when a situation calls for assertiveness, or you may uncover that you eat when you are tired and your body would prefer to go to bed. You may even learn that the urge to diet more rigorously may come from difficulty accepting a situation you cannot control.

The point is, when you judge your eating as "good" or "bad," you miss the valuable information that variations in your food choices can offer you. When you regain your freedom, you allow yourself to appreciate life's moments and are receptive to learning about yourself and your natural eating experiences. Suzanne's story illustrates how she changed her perception of a "bad day" to a "learning day":

> Suzanne had been enjoying satisfying eating experiences as a soulful eater when, for no apparent reason, she started to eat large amounts of food that made her physically uncomfortable. Because she was trying to understand her eating behavior instead of judging it she began to explore what feelings might be contributing to her desire to eat beyond her body's desires. When she did not reprimand herself for eating too much, as she had done in the past, she discovered her true feelings about a situation with a coworker. She felt her coworker was taking advantage of her, and she was angry with herself for allowing this to happen. Although she had been reluctant to disrupt the relationship with a confrontation, she realized it was time to express her feelings. She talked with her coworker and found that they could resolve their differences. Suzanne's willingness to learn from an eating pattern helped her uncover and resolve a lingering problem.

Self-Reflections

Questions to consider when choosing to eat:

What do you consider a "bad" eating day to be?

Next time you find yourself labeling a day as "bad" because of how you are eating, STOP yourself. Instead of writing it off as a "bad day," ask yourself the following questions: What is my eating pattern telling me about:

o *my body*—my physical needs and preferences?
o *my mind*—my thoughts and ideas?
o *my soul*—my innermost emotions, needs, and preferences?

DAILY REMINDER:

My body, mind, and soul have not had a chance to express their desires and needs through eating. I have cut off important information about my needs and desires by labeling certain kinds of eating as bad. Now I am ready to listen and learn. I will give my body a chance to teach me about some of its natural inclinations.

4. Let go of your dieting lifestyle. Eat what you want, when you want.

Exercise your freedom of choice. On a daily or hourly basis, think about what you *really* want to eat and then eat it. Do not try to figure out what you are *going* to want to eat next week or even tomorrow. Eat what you want *when* you want it. Have pizza for breakfast. Have cookies for lunch. Snack all day long if you feel like it, or eat only one big meal at night. If you crave a strange food, go ahead and eat it. When you do not find satisfaction in a meal, your food cravings may continue. Allow yourself the freedom to experiment as you begin to integrate your body, mind, and soul into your eating decisions.

Eating what you really want also includes *not eating* what you really do *not* want. If you do not want to eat anything at noon, then skip lunch. If you planned to have dessert but find yourself too full, pass it up. Or, you may eat a few bites of your dessert and leave the rest. You may leave food on your plate. If you ordered food but end up feeling too full to eat it, leave it or take it home. You may choose to skip any meal or planned snack if that feels natural to you at the time. You may discover that you do not want a piece of pie for dessert even though you are dining in a restaurant that has a reputation for great pie.

Perhaps you are not sure if you are hungry enough to have a second helping. Wait a few minutes and see how you feel. You can enjoy the social aspect of going out to pizza with friends even if you do not find yourself in the mood for eating pizza. You may decide not to eat a banquet meal that is unappealing to you and instead pick up a dinner that you really want on the way home. You may decide that although you are physically hungry, you are too tired to eat. If you realize that what you need is a little peace and quiet and not a piece of cake, skip the cake. The non-eating options in your soulful relationship with food are endless.

When you allow yourself to break free from the rules of dieting, your *best self* guides you to following your inner desires. In doing so, you open yourself to receiving and accepting life experiences that involve building a healthy relationship with food. In addition, by eliminating rules surrounding eating habits, you may also find that your body's natural cravings for adequate nutrition and healthy foods surface. If forbidden foods are no longer forbidden, and your body has free access to these foods, the desire for them diminishes significantly. The following eating experiences illustrate the importance of giving yourself the freedom to eat the way you wish.

Sheila went out to lunch with a definite desire for dessert. Since this was against her rules for losing weight, she ordered the salad bar and tried to satisfy her craving by eating two large salads with cheese, eggs, croutons, and dressing, and she also had potato salad, fruit salad, crackers, and bread. She consumed more fat and calories in her unsatisfying meal than if she had chosen the sandwich and dessert she had wanted so badly. Furthermore, her craving did not subside, and on her way home from the restaurant she bought three candy bars and ate them in her car.

Another client of mine found that after eating whatever she wanted for about three weeks, she began craving fruits and vegetables. She was surprised because these were foods she previously had to force herself to eat. One night she made a pizza and topped it with broccoli and mushrooms. She cut up some fruit and put it inside a crepe for dessert. It pleased her to have more interest in the fruit crepe than the chocolate cake that was still in her refrigerator.

Self-Reflections

Questions to consider when choosing to eat:

What factors currently determine what you are going to eat on a given day?

What decisions are already predetermined by weight control?

How much flexibility do you allow yourself in your daily eating choices? Do you allow for changes in your preferences, hunger level, emotions, plans and activities?

Allow yourself to explore what you really want to eat. Instead of going with a predetermined plan, STOP and ask yourself the following questions:

What sounds good to me right now?

What do I *really* want to eat?

How much do I want?

What will satisfy my true needs and desires right now?

DAILY REMINDER:

In deciding what I really want, I will consider my tastes, my hunger level, the texture and the availability of the food, my mood and any other variable EXCEPT *weight control.*

5. Expend energy according to your desires. Discover the pleasure in non-diet exercise for a healthful and enriching

living experience.

The method of choosing what you *really* want also applies to your decisions about physical exercise. Engage in physical activities because they appeal to you, not because you think you should. Do not engage in workouts for the main purpose of burning calories or burning fat. Go jogging if you want to experience the "runner's high." Join a dance class to socialize. If you want to release tension in the privacy of your own home, turn on your favorite music and dance around your living room. Use health clubs, ski clubs, ice skating, or walking your dog as methods to enhance your life with pleasurable experiences. Go for a walk or take a bike ride if you are in need of fresh air. If you were exercising solely for the purpose of weight loss, consider replacing it with a more satisfying activity. If you find that you would still like to continue the activity for other reasons, such as overall health benefits, focus on the enjoyment of your decision. Remember, however, that since you are no longer following a prescribed diet and exercise regime, you may choose the option to not exercise and not feel guilty. For example, Julie's following story shows how exercising, for reasons other than to lose weight, provided her with both emotional and physical satisfaction.

> Julie described her plan to go to her health club twice a week as a constant battle with herself. She stated that she felt proud after she forced herself to go, but often resented being inside the gym and cutting short the time she was able to spend outside. During one therapy session, Julie mentioned that she loved animals but did not have any pets of her own because of her husband's allergies. We discussed her option of volunteering at an

animal shelter to fulfill this desire. Within a few weeks, Julie had become an active volunteer. She walked dogs, cleaned kennels, carried bags of food and other supplies up and down stairs, and went to the health club less often. She even participated in a six-mile walk for the shelter's fundraiser. She gave up her health club membership and enjoyed spending more time outside participating in physical activities she thoroughly enjoyed.

Self-Reflections

Questions to consider for physical activities:

What physical exercises do you engage in?

What are your reasons for these exercises?

How do you feel about your exercise choices?

Which activities do you like? Which ones do you dislike?

What are physical activities you *really* enjoy? (If an answer does not come readily to mind, think about activities you enjoyed as a child or in your pre-diet days.)

What physical activities could you choose that also meet another desire?

    ○   *Do you want to meet new friends?*

o   *Do you want more time alone?*

o   *Do you want more time outside?*

o   *Do you want a competitive situation?*

o   *Do you want to learn a new skill?*

DAILY REMINDER:

Trust yourself self to make your own choices and revise them as you go. Allow flexibility in your decisions to engage in physical activities.

Best Self Eater vs. SAD Eater

The table on the following pages compares a day in the life of a *best self* eater to a day in the life of a SAD eater. Which kind of eater do you want to be?

COMPARISON OF A *BEST SELF* EATER'S DAY WITH THAT OF A SAD EATER		
TIME OF DAY	**JANE, THE SAD EATER**	**MARY, THE *BEST SELF* EATER**
7:00 am.	Jane awoke with the question "Will I be good today and stay on my diet?" She skipped breakfast, deciding to see how long she could go without eating. Jane brought rice cakes, a diet drink, and an apple with her to work.	"I have learned that I feel best when I eat breakfast," Mary said to herself as she began her day. While getting ready for work, she enjoyed the aroma of coffee brewing. On this cold winter day, she chose hot oatmeal with brown sugar and a sliced banana on top. She brought a bottle of water, her favorite crackers, and grapes with her to work.

8:30 a.m.	Jane arrived at work and saw that a coworker had brought doughnuts. Fearing that she might eat a doughnut, she tried to avoid them. The doughnuts were on her mind all day.	Mary's breakfast satisfied her and she had a productive morning at work.
10:30 am.	Jane could not resist. She cut a doughnut in half and quickly ate it. "I shouldn't have eaten it," she then said to herself.	During midmorning break, Mary discovered a coworker had brought homemade cinnamon rolls. While talking to her friends in the lounge and watching the snow fall, she ate grapes, drank half a cup of coffee, and enjoyed a small cinnamon roll.
NOON	Jane went to lunch reprimanding herself for eating half of the	Mary did not bring a lunch today because in the morning she could not decide what she

	doughnut. She decided to eat only a salad and a diet drink. Still hungry after eating the salad, she began eating the crackers from the breadbasket. She lost count and felt guilty. Although she was hungry, she was determined to make amends for the doughnut and crackers she thinks she should not have eaten.	would want. She and coworkers went to a cozy diner where she enjoyed soup, shared some French fries, and ate part of an egg salad sandwich.
2:30 p.m.	Because Jane was starving, she ate three fat-free rice cakes and an apple. She noticed there were two doughnuts remaining in the box, but they were not her favorite kind.	Mary, no longer hungry, found a quiet spot in a lounge near a window and sipped tea with lemon and honey from her favorite mug.

4:55 p.m.	Before leaving work, Jane impulsively grabbed the two leftover doughnuts and ate them as she walked to her car. She was upset because she had broken her diet and she vowed to do better tomorrow. Because her kitchen contained only diet food, she went to a fast-food drive-thru window and ordered two cheeseburgers, fries, and a shake. While driving home, she ate the meal quickly.	Unwinding in her favorite chair, Mary satisfied her hunger by munching on carrots and crackers. She then carefully decided what she would like to eat. She selected her grandmother's bread pudding for dessert because it brought back fond childhood memories. She had no other obvious cravings, so she made a vegetable stir-fry and warmed some fresh bakery bread. She set the table, lit a candle, played classical music, and ate dinner.

9:00 p.m.	Jane munched on "diet food" all evening. Without thinking, she began to eat handfuls of cereal directly from the box. She finished the fat-free yogurt intended to be three entire meals according to her diet. She ate the remaining rice cakes. Deriving little enjoyment from this food and feeling sick, Jane wrote out her plan for tomorrow, consisting of a strict diet and rigorous exercise.	Later that evening Mary called her grandmother for a short chat before eating her bread pudding. They enjoyed a pleasant conversation and reminisced about a time when Mary and her grandmother were snowbound together for two days and feasted on bread pudding.

CHAPTER III

STEP 3: INFORMING

Becoming Informed, Not Programmed

The third step to finding your unique connection with food is to choose what *you* want to know about your body, mind, and soul, your deepest self, and what you would like to find out about the food options that are available. As your inner wisdom reclaims its position as your guide in your soulful journey with food, the process of becoming *informed,* not *programmed,* unfolds. SAD diets tell you what to eat and what not to eat and how to try harder if you fail to adhere to its rules. This dict-based, weight loss-focused "knowledge" may have become so ingrained within you that you have come to view these inner struggles as a normal part of your relationship with food. These conflicts created by a false understanding of yourself and food, however, are actually blocking your ability to hear the expressions of your soul, your deepest essence. This obstructing information needs to be deprogrammed so it stops influencing your approach to food.

As you remove your diet mask created by SAD thinking, the false beliefs you have had about your relationship with food will be replaced with an under-standing of the deeper needs and desires of your soul. At times, these discoveries may be more challenging to face than a structured diet, but as Authenticity, Acceptance, and Appreciation direct your relationship with food, a peaceful relationship with food and a deeper quality of all life experiences will unfold for you. The following table offers ways that you can identify your soul's true expression as you let go of the obstructing thoughts and behaviors created by SAD.

SAD Thought	Soul's Expression
False control	Letting Go
Overeating	Fulfilling
Starving	Striving
Blowing It	Going with it
Failing	Feeling
Measuring	Treasuring
Preoccupation	Inspiration
Dieting	Living

Replace *False Control* with *Letting Go*

Do you feel a sense of purpose when following a diet? One of life's valuable lessons is learning to distinguish between what is within your control and what is not. Dieting offers an escape from facing this lesson by providing a general illusion of control. When you allow your level of success with your diet to set your mood and your sense of accomplishment—even your self-worth—you are giving your diet a false control over your life. If you are feeling vulnerable in other areas of your life you may even try to increase your sense of control through dieting.

When you stop hiding behind the rules of dieting you will face the struggle of understanding the limits of what you can control. You may experience disappointment when you try to change a situation that is not within your control. But, ultimately, it is important to feel the frustration that may be present and learn to let go. Authentic acceptance of what you cannot alter will replace false ideas of invincibility and you will find peace. Mary's experience illustrates her use of diet beliefs to try to gain a false sense of control:

> Mary struggled with her husband's inability to voice his feelings of love for her. She became convinced early in the relationship that if she lost weight he would find her more lovable and would then express his affections. Dieting tricked her into believing that her actions could affect her husband's emotional issues. She did not consider his inability to express love or her need to receive affection from him. It was easier for her to believe that they would live "happily ever after" if her body were a few sizes smaller. What Mary did not consider was that perhaps her husband's inability to

express his emotions was much more deeply rooted than Mary's appearance. Mary continued to believe that the relationship was completely in her hands and would be fixed as soon as she dieted successfully. Mary's *best self* wanted her to ask the following questions: Is this marriage satisfying? Can I accept not having verbal expressions of love from my husband but enjoy his other signs of love? What is the best way to discuss these feelings with my husband? Can he help me understand his verbal inhibitions? Will he try to change? Struggling with these questions rather than her weight would have led Mary to a more helpful understanding of herself, her husband, and their relationship.

Replace *Overeating* with *Fulfilling*

Do you overeat to the point of physical discomfort? One of the most common dieting experiences is overeating. When your body is in a semi-starved state it is a normal physiological reaction to overeat when given the chance. Furthermore, when dieting overeating may occur as an attempt to "stuff" your feelings, to distract yourself from your emotional needs and desires. When your body recognizes that it is semi-starved you may end up eating foods high in fat and sugar very rapidly if given the chance. As a result, you feel stuffed. Then you feel ashamed because you broke your diet. Your solution is to increase your food restrictions and ignore your hunger, which will only lead to more episodes of overeating. This scenario is familiar to many dieters.

Overeating may be your body's attempt to become less deprived, combined with your soul's way of expressing an internal emptiness. Perhaps you want some love, some nurturing, or just some time to yourself. Maybe you need to vent some anger or cry over a situation that did not go the way you had planned. Your inner self may be asking you to recognize a difficult dilemma that will continue to cause a void in your life until you resolve it. If you can listen to the message beneath overeating rather than condemn the behavior, you can discover what you really need to find for fulfillment. Jill's following experience shows how she attempted to satisfy her internal needs by eating too much:

> Jill felt trapped in a cycle of overeating episodes that were escalating in frequency. After bingeing, she would become disgusted with herself and feel undeserving of happiness. She chose to punish herself by limiting social outings and fun activities. Her soul continued to express its emptiness through her habit of overeating and Jill continued to punish herself rather than listen to the message from within. When Jill stopped punishing herself and engaged in more social activities, she satisfied the true need for friendship that her *best self* was trying to tell her about, and with her newfound companionship the overeating and the desire to binge diminished.

Replace *Starving* with *Striving*

Do you sometimes enjoy the famished feeling in your stomach and intentionally refuse to eat when your body is sending you signals that it needs food? Weight loss-focused eating produces not only the desire to overeat but also the desire to intentionally starve yourself. Have you ever felt especially strong and energetic during times when you have eaten barely anything? Perhaps you associate a flattened belly, an empty feeling, and growling in your stomach with a sense of accomplishment and achievement. Have you felt powerful when you have been able to fight normal physical signals to eat? Perhaps you have felt embarrassingly pleased when someone hears your grumbling stomach. Intellectually, you may recognize that starving is ineffective as a long-term method for obtaining a sense of accomplishment, but it feels good to be able to brag about how long you have gone without eating.

Your soul may be expressing your need to recognize a neglected desire or to make a challenging choice. Preoccupation with dieting is masking this awareness since the feeling of starvation is challenging and feels like a step toward a desired goal; however, from the *best self*'s viewpoint, starving is irrelevant to accomplishment and does not result in long-term weight loss or a sense of purpose. A meaningful desire that reaffirms your sense of purpose lies beneath the starving act. The process of striving for authenticity, unlike starving, is truly energizing, invigorating, and motivating. My client Lois learned how to replace starving with striving:

> Although Louis worked hard in hopes of getting a job promotion, her efforts went unnoticed and unappreciated. Lois soon found herself skipping breakfast and lunch on her workdays, believing that her concentration improved and her energy increased when she did not eat. She hoped this would lead to more attention and recognition and, ultimately, a promotion. However, not eating all day was not in any way related to advancement in her job. This false sense of achieving through starving also masked her intuitive feeling that she would need to change jobs to obtain a higher

position. It was only when she began eating breakfast and lunch again that Lois realized her strong need to be elevated to a position with more responsibility required either a confrontation with her boss or looking for a different job.

Replace *Blowing It* with *Going with It*

Do you feel angry with yourself when you go off your diet? Have you ever said, "I'm blowing my diet" when you eat something from your forbidden list or eat more food than you had allowed? Have you ever had a "good week" and then found you were eating uncontrollably and "blowing it" afterward? Once this happens do you continue eating large amounts of unsatisfying food, vowing to do better tomorrow?

Your inner voice is protesting the eating rules and restrictions you have imposed. Your *best self* does not want you to feel content with a diet that is interfering with more important things in life. It does not want you to feel proud because you ate under twelve hundred calories. Your soul wants you to consider the emotional and physical needs that may be contributing to different kinds of eating. You can learn more about your bodily needs by accepting and exploring your actions than by simply labeling your behavior as "bad." Contrary to what the diet world preaches, you are expressing a courageous strength in this act of diet rebellion. Your innermost self is trying to become free from the diet trap. "Blowing it" is really a sign that a wiser part of you knows that dieting is interfering with your ability to enjoy life. "Going with it" may result in new insights about your eating preferences, an awareness of a masked emotion, or a deeper understanding of a conflict. Or, it may simply mean having to accept an unexplainable eating episode. For example, I think of Anita, who came to her first therapy session feeling confused and dejected:

> Anita felt proud of herself for sticking to a strict diet and losing weight, although it was consuming most of her time and energy. She expressed feeling anxious over a craving for a cheeseburger that she tried to satisfy with a rice cake and a salad. The next thing she knew she was fast food hopping and she ate burgers from three different places. In addition, she had French fries and a milk shake—food items she rarely craved. She described feeling as if "someone else was in charge of my hands and shoveling in the food as fast as they could." Anita felt unhappy about "blowing it" and vowed to resume her diet the next day, hoping a few therapy sessions might strengthen her ability to diet. While presenting the idea of "going with it," I suggested that Anita's body might have been craving protein because her current diet allowed very little food of substance. Furthermore, her spirit might be rebelling against spending so much time on her diet rather than tending to other interesting parts of her life. She seemed relieved to consider the option of getting off the diet and "going with it" while exploring other personal issues.

Replace *Failing* with *Feeling*

Do you ever describe yourself as a failed dieter? Given that more than a ninety-five percent failure rate in maintaining weight loss follows diets, most individuals engaged in rule-bound eating have experienced diet failure. Even when you know the statistics do you blame yourself when you fail and still want to be able to complete a restricted eating regimen? Your perception of yourself as a failure probably results in a renewed or even stronger commitment to your next diet. This stubborn conviction sets you up for a downfall when the new dieting program's promise is also unfulfilled.

Your soul may be asking you to look at other feelings rather than focusing on the weight gain or the extra food intake. You may be disappointed in yourself for reasons unrelated to weight control. Your soul may be asking for forgiveness, self-acceptance, or a change to take place in your life. *Weight loss is not success and weight gain is not failure.* Dieting is not a rewarding lifestyle, even if you do lose weight. Michelle and her story about her first successful diet can best illustrate this concept:

> Michelle remembered thinking it was "so easy to lose weight" that she believed anyone who tried hard enough should be able to do it. When she dieted, she woke up with her eating plan on her mind every morning and went to bed with thoughts about food every night. Oblivious to the things that were happening in the world around her, she was succeeding on a diet. Then she experienced a few weeks of "cheating" on her diet. Michelle told me her "willpower was slipping, and the pounds were inching back on." She focused on her feelings of failure and tried everything she could to regain a sense of accomplishment. Michelle realized that she was holding on to the feeling of diet failure to avoid acceptance of her daughter's recently diagnosed disability. When she began to accept the confusion and sadness she felt about her daughter's condition and began to explore the options, dieting for success or

failure became irrelevant.

Replace *Measures* with *Treasures*

Diets rely on measuring devices. Scales are the first line of defense, measuring rates of success in pounds. Skin calipers measure the percentage of body fat. Measuring is also used to count calories, carbohydrates, or grams of fat. How do you measure your success? Do you use a scale, a tape measure, or a clothing size for evaluation? Do you weigh yourself at least once a week, daily, or even hourly? Is getting on the scale a ritual for you? If you are a part of a group weight loss program, you may be familiar with going hungry the night before an official weigh-in and then overeating afterward. Do you feel regret and anxiety about eating after a "bad" weigh-in? Do you feel a sense of accomplishment after a "good" weigh-in or other signs of weight loss? Do you consult books that list the contents of food items? Do you spend significant time planning your food intake and measuring your food into portions?

Your soul wants you to treasure yourself and appreciate who you are. Your worthiness does not depend on your body size and your ability to change it through artificially prescribed procedures. Rather than counting inches your soul is asking you to value your unique self and admire your strength in handling an emergency or solving a conflict diplomatically. Your soul wants you to praise your ability to laugh at yourself and cherish your gifts for listening, singing, making mistakes, and learning. Cultivate the ability to see that eating struggles may signal a need for self-appreciation rather than self-evaluation.

In addition to self-appreciation, treasure your food

choices rather than analyze them according to their calorie content. Savor food for its ability to contribute to soulful living. The practice of "treasuring" may include a day of baking cookies with a child or a friend, sharing the cookie dough, and together eating the first batch of hot cookies right out of the oven. The values of your interactions with food include your ability to enjoy taste, have preferences, react to texture, and enjoy your meals without guilt. When you acknowledge the gift of a healthy appetite you fulfill the desire to nourish both body and soul. Margie recently expressed the joy of giving up dieting as she replaced measures with treasures, as expressed in the following example:

> When Margie told me, "I was abusing my body with binges and purges. I did unhealthy things just to see the right numbers on the scale! Life was passing me by. I'm thankful that it is not too late for me to appreciate my health, my body, and the way I eat. I am truly blessed to have a body that I can feed and to have wonderful food available to nurture it!" Margie rediscovered the abundance in her life that was hidden by her obsession with dieting and losing weight and has continued on her path of allowing her inner wisdom to guide her relationship with food.

Replace *Preoccupation* with *Inspiration*

Do you become obsessed with food and dieting? Do you get caught up in the wave of losing weight and become preoccupied with the details of menu planning and exercising? Do your conversations center on the details of a diet? Do you forego attending certain events to avoid the presence of tempting foods?

Concentrating on eating rules and restrictions consumes energy when you make them a central part of your daily life. Do you list, graph, or chart your weight-loss progress? Do you plaster diet rules on the refrigerator? Does this narrow focus on food regulations and limitations dictate your thoughts and your activities?

Your soul may be looking for a way to express itself. Although your preoccupation may offer the security of having rules to follow, it interferes with creative inspiration. Your spontaneous ideas cannot find expression when you are obsessing over eating programs and body size. Leave the door open for insight from your *best self* to come forward at any time. It may appear as a humorous response, a sudden hunch, or even a flash of instinctual wisdom. Whatever form it may take, it is important for you to be aware of the information your *best self* is trying to provide you with. I am reminded of John, a client who had some new ideas for reorganizing his small business:

> John could see that the inefficient procedures in his present office layout demoralized his employees. John was also a dieter and put detailed constraints on his eating choices. He had arranged his apartment to make room for exercise equipment and he used colorful charts and journals to measure his weight loss progress. His refrigerator and cupboards were arranged based on meal plans. John often came home at night prepared to work on the restructuring of his office, but would spend his evening developing new diet plans and meal schemes instead. His organizational ability was consumed with dieting and he was never able to apply this skill to his office. Once John freed himself from his preoccupation with dieting he discovered several new

ideas for his business. His new layout improved office morale, his business showed growth, and John experienced more satisfaction. By allowing his spontaneous insight some room to grow, he nourished the essence of his being and applied his natural gifts to developing a comfortable and efficient work atmosphere. He now enjoys the benefits of a pleasant work environment and the structured eating regimens that he struggled to adhere to at home have ended.

Replace *Dieting* with *Living*

Does dieting feel like your way of life? Does SAD detract from the quality of your day-to-day existence? Do the natural experiences of everyday life take a back seat to diet demands? Have you lost days, weeks, or even years to measuring, obsessing, and controlling?

Your soul wants a chance to lead you to the unlimited abundance of life. When you conduct your life ignoring your innermost needs, you deprive your true self from experiencing the fullness of being alive. One of my clients expressed her excitement about her new natural approach to eating when she described her life of dieting as "living on hold" and said she already felt like her new soulful approach was opening up a whole new world for her.

No longer masked with programmed information from a weight loss-focused lifestyle, you will instinctually seize the chance to explore your true self, discover more of what life has to offer you, and find new meaning and mystery in your everyday experiences. You have now made room for your *best self* to use all of its wisdom as it takes in both intuitive knowledge and acquired information about you and about food in creating each eating experience and integrating it into the flow of your life each day.

A Return to the Natural Way through Intuitive Information

Your *best self* listens to intuitive information from your body, mind, and soul as it interacts with all that life is presenting. What does *best self* intuition look like?

Our bodies tell us what they need if we are willing to listen and to respond. One of my workshop participants reported that since she is more attuned to what her natural food desires are, she has stronger desires for steamed broccoli and green beans. A vegetarian who used to excessively count fat grams reported that when she craves peanut butter she now knows it is a signal that she needs more protein and doesn't resist eating it. Another ex-dieter noted that she naturally wants fruit and juice when she has a cold. She believes this is her body's way of asking for vitamin C. Because these people have rid themselves of external rules about food they are in touch with their physical needs on a daily basis. Without thought, our bodies will naturally tell us when they have had enough fat or sugar. Ex-SAD eaters have told me that they sometimes eat only part of their dessert, or that they no longer have the desire to consume a whole bag of potato chips or a box of cookies. They have found that when they listen to what their bodies need they feel satisfied and energized. People enjoying the freedom of making their own food choices one experience at a time are surprised to discover that some of the sugary or high-fat foods that were hardest for them to resist while dieting have now lost their appeal and they rarely crave them.

Gathering intuitive information may include taking note of the taste of your favorite foods, recognizing a sweet aroma from the past, or being in the company of family and friends at dinner. We rediscover the enjoyment of preparing a meal that we desire. We choose foods that might bring up a fond memory or provide comfort in a particularly stressful time. An intuitive choice might be to reward yourself after a busy morning at work by taking the time to eat your favorite lunch. The intuitive knowledge that a refreshing Italian ice or an ice cream cone with your kids on a hot summer afternoon may lead you to a satisfying trip to the ice cream parlor and the creation of a special memory for all of you. An insistent desire for pizza may reflect a deep longing for a carefree evening out with friends, with or without the pizza. When we listen intuitively we embrace our cravings as a valuable expression to explore rather than as an indulgent urge to resist, and in turn we enrich our everyday living.

A Return to the Natural Way through Acquired Information

Becoming informed, rather than programmed, can be a challenge. Socially Acceptable Deprivation (SAD) has us looking for information that tells us what, when, and how much to eat. Even when we do not actively seek it we are constantly bombarded with information designed for the weight loss-focused consumer. A wide range of structured eating plans try to convince us that they know the best way for us to eat based on their analysis of the scientific properties of certain foods and supplements. Some programs involve complicated formulas and calculations in preparing a meal while others present information to convince you that you only need to buy their pre-made packages. I personally recall trying to follow a diet that required special food combinations at certain times and I remember being afraid that consuming just one olive could alter the magic chemistry that promised quick weight loss. Perhaps you unknowingly are letting a lifetime accumulation of facts about food related to weight loss, such as calories, carbohydrates, and fat grams, determine your eating choices. But now that the goal of weight loss is no longer the criteria for deciding what you are going to eat or not eat ask yourself what information you want to discard and what other kind of knowledge you would like to acquire and consider when contemplating food choices.

No book, including this one, can provide you with specific instructions about what foods you should eat and how and when you should eat them. That would interfere with your discovery of your unique relationship with food. Only your *best self* should be in charge of the way you use the information that you already have about food and the decision to gather new information. Understanding your particular preferences as to how, when, and what you eat and exploring how these choices affect your overall wellbeing is up to you.

Self-Reflections
Acquiring Information about You

What kind of information about yourself would you like to explore when creating each eating experience? What knowledge about you as an eater will help you make your lifelong relationship with food all that you want it to be?

Your eating style may vary every day or you may find that there are certain consistencies in the way you prefer to eat that reveal your uniqueness. Knowledge about you and your preferences is the key to understanding what eating experiences will create a peaceful and natural relationship with food for you. Look within. Take in information about where and when you prefer to eat as well as your preferences based on who you uniquely are.

Authentic preferences include choices about where you like to eat, whether it's at home or out. When at home you may find that you may be in the mood to sit down to a formally set table at times, and eating from paper plates on the deck or patio may be your preference at other times. Do you prefer a table, the bar, the booth, the car, or a picnic table when the choice to eat out is made? As you anticipate going out, is an old favorite restaurant what you need to relax and unwind or does the thought of a new adventure in eating speak to your desires?

While diets often set up a rigid time schedule that informs the dieter when to eat, *best self* eating has unlimited possibilities. Authentic information may include that you enjoy eating three meals a day or that you are a person who likes to graze on small amounts all day long. You may find comfort in establishing eating routines or your eating style could change daily. Allow the choices to reveal your present life's true expressions. A late night pizza with old friends from college who happen to be driving through town may require you to eat later than preferred, but is a choice that offers spontaneous fun and conviviality.

Becoming deprogrammed means allowing your

best self to explore the wide range of eating experiences including ways that you enjoyed food before you ever imposed a rule. Perhaps you enjoy a sweet treat after dinner as you experienced in childhood. Or is there a particular way that you ate as a child that you now realize is not part of your natural style? My client, Molly, describes one of her consistent comforts of childhood was Sunday morning family breakfast. She recalls waking up in the morning to the familiar enticing aromas coming from the kitchen. Molly enjoys continuing her family tradition of a full Sunday morning breakfast; the smells, the bustling in the kitchen, and the decorated table with all the place settings and accouterments speak to her authentic nature. My client, Patty, however, experienced her Sunday morning family breakfasts in childhood as a delay to pursuing her desires for the day and as an adult, she finds a quick on-the-go breakfast to be her true preference the majority of the time. The key is to understand what your true desires are when creating your own eating experiences.

In addition to revisiting information about your eating preferences before you were programmed by SAD, understanding your present preferences may be worth considering as you create eating experiences aligned with your true nature. In working with so many people with differing eating styles over the years, I have found that knowing what kind of eater you are makes it easier to make satisfying choices. For example, there are people who I refer to as "bulk eaters" who feel most satisfied when large amounts of food are present in the meal. Knowing that this is one's preference will ensure many fulfilling eating experiences. For example, the "bulk eater" is likely to prefer a large bowl of popcorn over one small piece of rich chocolate candy. Persons with this preference enjoy a plate piled high with salads and veggies more than just a half of a sandwich. Furthermore, they prefer a variety of food choices available to them when they sit down to eat, even though they may not choose to eat it all. In a similar vein, there are those who like to experiment with new foods and different ways to eat and others who are most content with certain kinds of food that they consider to be their staples. Then there are those individuals sensitive to specific tastes and anything less than meeting those desires are not satisfying. For example, an individual with this preference may know that eating fresh fruit from a farm stand is the only way that they enjoy peaches and apples. Or perhaps, for these individuals, nothing short of real butter and pure maple syrup on their pancakes will give them the satisfaction of a good old-fashioned breakfast.

Acquiring Information about Food

While knowledge obtained solely for the purpose of losing weight obstructs the natural way, learning about the qualities of food that apply to *your* unique style offers experiences that fulfill body, mind, and soul. Seek information that matters to *you* rather than simply listening to another newsflash or fad as to what you should be eating or not eating for your health. One place to start is to stop accepting as "truth" what food labels describe as "healthy" or what the diet community judges as "unhealthy." Consider taking the time to understand the true nutritional value of food items that you already enjoy rather than simply accepting a persuasive marketing strategy to eat food that holds little appeal to you.

Instead of counting calories or grams of fat, you may want to consider information about your body's nutritional needs. Would you like to become familiar with the basic nutritional values of fruits and vegetables, grains and fiber, protein, and decreased saturated fats? Do you want to find out about minerals and vitamins and their role in maintaining a healthy body? What satisfies your tastes, fulfills your senses, and still provides what your body needs? Think of the information you are gathering as being a contribution to the options that the *best self* considers when choosing what to eat. Perhaps you would enjoy acquiring new knowledge about food that is available to eat by going grocery shopping in some new places. Try farm stands, co-ops, cooking classes, health food stores, and perhaps even some interesting websites. Learn about food characteristics relevant to your physical needs, but be sure to include your taste preferences in your investigation. Select foods you have never tried but find yourself drawn to or curious about after exploring new options. Can you increase your time grocery shopping, browsing farmer's markets, or preparing meals? Are you willing to spend a little more money on food if necessary?

Acquiring Information about You and Food Together

What do you know about your family history as it might relate to the properties of food? You may discover a pattern suggesting a physical vulnerability or predisposition to a medical condition that will give you an opportunity to avoid health problems in the future that seem to correlate to certain eating patterns. Consider having a physical examination or other kinds of evaluations offered by physicians or alternative health providers. Be aware that some of the medical experts' positions on weight loss may not be consistent with *best self* eating. You are not looking for a prescribed diet, pills, or surgery. Forget the illusions of the "quick fix" diet; consider taking input from a medical intuitive, chiropractor, naturopath, acupuncturist, or other alternative holistic approaches to health that appeal to you. Experts in food and health may have viewpoints that your *best self* may want to consider at varying times in your life as you make food choices that fulfill your whole person, body, mind, and soul.

Go ahead and explore any information that comes your way that may be pertinent to your relationship with food. Keep in mind that you are simply getting a collection of many different viewpoints obtained in many different ways. We have all experienced the changing nature of "facts" when it comes to food and eating. Foods that might be held up as "good for you" one year may fall to the "bad for you" list by the following year. Don't be afraid to explore any new information. Don't take it too seriously either. Even if you believe that adhering to some of the new ideas could be beneficial to you, remember that they are not rules or obligations.

For good or for bad, the current state of technology allows almost any piece of information or question that you might have to be right at your fingertips. We are truly in an age of information and it is more important than ever to realize we do not have to become prisoners to it, but rather we can use it to better our lives in our own way. You may want to watch a video on the influence of our food and exercise choices on the prevention of heart attacks, cancer, and many other diseases and physical ailments. Information about the role of food in allergies, diabetes, inflammation, and chronic pain may hold some interest to you. After reading the benefits of a detoxification or weekly fasting, some people choose to try it. Freed from the restrictions that are based on weight loss-focused eating, new eaters sometimes choose to set guidelines for what categories of food they are going to eat and others they might be more inclined to avoid. I have a friend who no longer diets but enjoys the parameters that she has chosen to set herself instead, an eating style that she believes enhances her health and wellbeing. She avoids oils, refined sugars, and processed food. She keeps plenty of fruits and vegetables readily available. She describes herself as feeling more comfortable with these parameters because they feel like helpful guidelines for grocery shopping and making daily choices about eating. My friend finds it easier to eat the way she really wants to with these boundaries in place and experiences no sense of being restricted, limited, or deprived.

Information may come your way about the effects of our food choices on the suffering of animals or the environment. My vegan preference began when I learned about what typically is involved with factory farming at the same time that I became more aware of my sensitivity to and concern with the plight of animals. Likewise, you may find that new information combined with your personal values may result in a significant change in the way you eat, but your new decisions will flow easily because they are the natural result of wanting to make choices that are aligned with your values. Some information that you acquire will give you additional insight into what physiological factors might be influencing some of your eating choices. For example, there is research that suggests the brain, as an organ of the body, can become physically addicted to sugar and dairy products. An awareness of this information may shed a different light on how you view your cravings and choose to consume those products. I know people who decided to not eat refined sugar and dairy for two weeks and have experienced the dissipation of those intense cravings for that kind of food, as the findings suggest. You may want to try it or you may not. Acquiring information does not obligate you to any action except those that you choose to do. Take it in and allow a whole new world of you and food to open!

DAILY REMINDER:

I am only gaining knowledge. There is no obligation to act on what I discover. Information that pertains to me will increase rather than constrict my freedom of choice as I expand my understanding of my options.

CHAPTER IV

STEP 4: DECIDING

Trusting the Decision-Making Process

Let the fun begin! The fourth step on your new journey is learning to trust the instinctive decision-making process of your innermost wisdom. Remember that a natural relationship with food that integrates itself peacefully into your everyday life is already within you. Your *best self* is ready to respond each time you decide to eat and ask yourself "What eating experience do I want now?" It is the last two words of this question—"want" and "now"—that invite your inner wisdom to direct your eating experiences. "Want" refers to the desires of your whole person—body, mind, and soul. "Now" means "in the present moment," that is what you want without the thought system that you have carried in the past and without the focus of the outcome of weight loss that has kept you in the future—just right now. The Three As—Authenticity, Acceptance, and Appreciation—are then able to direct each decision with ease as our natural relationship with food has a chance to play out, one eating experience at a time.

Want

Perhaps your reaction to the idea of eating what you want is similar to many skeptical dieters' and you might ask the following: If I allow my desires to enter the picture, won't I eat a cheeseburger and fries every night for dinner and cake and candy all day? And the answer is simple: No. Those scenarios are more likely to happen when we do not take into account the desires of the whole person. Your *best self* considers the desires of your body, mind, and soul when making a decision and does not respond only to one craving, an urge that was most likely intensified by the SAD thought that these choices are forbidden. Eating only candy all day or fast food at night would be ignoring your body's natural desire for nutrition and so that would not be a daily choice of your inner wisdom. Remember that you are listening to what you want from a new, deeper place and you no longer have the artificially induced desire of wanting something that you are not allowed to have. With the exception of a life-threatening food allergy or other health condition, no choice is forbidden. There may be times that you eat too many sweets and don't nourish your body with the nutrition that it needs to work best on any given day, but you can trust that your inner wisdom has its own self-correcting mechanism in place. When allowed to function without the self-defeating thoughts of guilt and failure overindulgence in one meal will result in a natural adjustment in another.

It may seem hard to believe that you could really trust yourself in such a way, but look at how you handle other non-food related areas of your life where differing desires emerge for reassurance. For example, there may be a part of us that sometimes wants to stay in bed all day. Perhaps on occasion we indulge ourselves and do just that. On most mornings, however, we automatically sort through *all* of our needs and desires: the urge to stay in bed, the sense of responsibility to show up at work, and the need to stimulate our minds and be productive. Usually, with little extra effort, we decide to get up and start the day. Likewise, our *best selves* consider all of our needs and desires in the moment when we make food choices. We simply have forgotten to trust it when it comes to our relationship with food.

The following situations, described by workshop participants, illustrate the possibility of choices that can take place when inner wisdom accepts differing concerns of the body, mind, and soul and finds ways to integrate them into a *best self* eating experience.

> Maria loved to cook and bake, but because one of her children was allergic to eggs and dairy products she felt limited in the recipes she could use. Besides the inconvenience, Maria noticed that her cravings for eggs and dairy were often not satisfied because she preferred not to serve them in front of her child who couldn't digest them. With a little creativity, however, she was able to satisfy her own cravings while enjoying family meals together by finding tasty dairy and egg substitutes such as soymilk, pumpkin, and apple butter that satisfied her preferences. She tried a variety of nondairy desserts made with almond, soy, and coconut milks and, to her delightful surprise, she discovered an alternative that she now prefers to her previously favorite ice cream.
>
> Susan talked about an eating experience she had while

exploring her natural cravings. One hot summer day she acknowledged her urge for some kind of refreshing dessert. Her all-time favorite was a turtle sundae: vanilla ice cream, caramel sauce, hot fudge, pecans, and whipped cream. She identified her desire for something tasty to cool and refresh her. She considered the option of the previously forbidden turtle sundae, but surprisingly realized that was not her first choice in this moment. She really wanted two scoops of Italian ice and when she chose it she knew she had made the perfect choice in responding to her craving. Susan's decision had nothing to do with the fact that Italian ice has less fat and calories than ice cream; a turtle sundae continues to be an option she is free to choose when considering refreshing desserts.

These two stories illustrate the freedom of choice that is available to the *best self* in the decision-making process. Rule-bound eating restricts your decision-making process. When satisfying a craving means that you are eating outside of the rules you were to follow, a programmed response of self-defeat, guilt, and feelings of failure are likely to occur. Flexibility, compromise, and creativity are blocked by the belief that you gave in to a desire that you needed to ignore. The key to freedom is to not run your desires through the structure of the artificial thought system formed by SAD. Instead listen to the many facets of your body, mind, and soul all interacting together to explore endless choices, arriving at a decision that creates the eating experience that is best at that moment. Can you let your inner wisdom flow without the rules and without the focus on an outcome based on weight loss? When you trust yourself to consider *all* of the options in that moment and come to your own decisions, however, you accept the possibility that choices can vary from day to day, even from hour to hour. You already allow your inner wisdom to guide you in other areas of your life. It's just a matter of bringing that same level of trust to your food choices.

Think about your approach to sleeping. We all know that it is important to get enough sleep, yet most of us do not adhere to a strict sleep schedule. It is unlikely that you have followed one set of rules about sleep throughout your life. Perhaps you have stayed up late to take care of a baby, write a paper, or extend an enjoyable evening. You accept the natural consequences of lack of sleep, like feeling tired and irritable or being less efficient. You might make a conscious decision to go to bed early the next day, or you may find yourself falling asleep while reading the paper. You are free to live with what happens when you do not get enough sleep and continue to make choices about sleep. It is helpful to approach eating in a similar way. Just as you allow the priority you give to the need for rest to vary, depending on what is happening, so, too, can you naturally allow variations in your eating patterns.

Now

When you recognize that the present moment is really all that you ever have and all that you ever need you are able to fully live life—one moment at a time. You will realize that any information needed by your inner wisdom to make a decision is available to you, including the choices you make to create your eating experiences. You simply need to listen from deep within, the place where your natural relationship with food already lies. It is beneath and beyond all the thoughts of the past and future that take you away from the present moment. When you leave the past behind, you also abandon the labels that you may have for yourself that try to influence your choices. Self-descriptors you may use include *overeater*, *stress-eater*, *binge-eater*, *dieter*, *food addict*, or a person with poor willpower. You will also let go of the obstructing thoughts that you attach to food, like words such as *temptations*, *forbidden food*, *triggers*, *bad food*, *wrong food,* or items that you should or shouldn't eat. And along with these labels you can go even further and dismiss those thoughts that define your interactions with food, like "If I eat *x*, then *y* will happen," or conclusions that you will draw about yourself if you make a certain choice, like thoughts about your wavering willpower. Patterns and habits of the past belong exactly there—in the past. For example, you are at the movies and you hear yourself say, "I always have popcorn at the movies." You know that is an option you can take, but instead of automatically ordering it make sure you ask yourself that important question: What eating experience do I want now? Do you really want popcorn or is it an automatic response because it is a treat you allow when dieting? This is a new moment and your response does not have to be influenced by what you did the last time you were at the movies. The idea is the same for wedding cake and birthday cake or food at baseball games. Yes, you have the choice to eat any of it, but you can also decide to enjoy the events without it. Past choices, habits, and restrictions are not helpful to think about as you approach each fresh moment at hand. They block all that is possible *right now*, including eating in a way that doesn't even resemble how you used to eat. Everything is possible in the new moment. New moments allow free access to that natural relationship with food that already resides within you.

Likewise, the beliefs that you carry about how you should eat to achieve an outcome in the future must also be left at the door. When eating in the present you are no longer eating to achieve an outcome in the future. Even those images of yourself when you were thinner that you thought were inspiring actually detract from the decision process of your *best self.* You are assessing everything that is right now before you and choosing the best eating experience with the vast amount of information that is immediately available to you—right there.

In directing each eating experience, your *best self* will naturally allow the Three As to guide its decision-making process right at that moment:

Authenticity

Take in information about yourself without judgment. Notice your mood, your tastes, and your body's needs. Play with the possibilities. Discover yourself as you relate to food. You might overeat. You might not eat enough. You might eat only one large meal in a given day and seven small meals on another. Go with it. Play with it. Enjoy. Learn. Allow yourself to undergo all of your feelings, even those you would rather not have. Listen fully to what you know about you right now—and accept it. You may find that, one moment at a time, you seem to prefer to not eat late at night. You might find that you feel better not eating dairy products. You may find that certain decisions regarding food choices seem to be more aligned with other values that you choose to not eat food based on who you are—and they don't feel like restrictions, they feel like the real you.

Acceptance

Now take in the information that is outside of you in the moment and accept whatever that might be without judgment. *Accept* compromises, mistakes, and varying situations in life. Accept that what you thought you wanted this moment to be, isn't. But it's okay just the way it is. Acceptance comes into play when the situation around you doesn't hold the option that your *best self* came up with for eating. Perhaps there is a food that you would rather not eat, but you also don't want to hurt the person's feelings who went through the trouble of making it for you. That's a choice. Maybe you are just too hungry to wait until you have a chance to get home and make what you really want and find a less desirable option. You may know this and are not surprised when it is not as satisfying.

Appreciation

Appreciate the ups and downs of life and the ups and downs of eating. Understand the complexities of your relationship with food. If you are making a decision that is not based on the past and not considering the future, it might feel strange. Just go with it and see where it leads. It doesn't have to be a heavy matter. Take it lightly and enjoy it. There's always another moment to make a different choice.

Your *best self* will then make its best choice in that moment. It's simply responding to the natural, best relationship that you have with food that is already there. Asking yourself, "What eating experience do I want now?" alerts your *best self* to respond, but even when you don't feel like asking yourself the question you can continue to trust your inner wisdom to make the most of each eating experience.

TAKE ACTION:
Make the Decision to Eat

Before you begin to eat, take a little time to quiet your thoughts so you are truly in a position to listen deeply to what the desires of your mind, body, and soul might be. Sense your feelings and intuition. Listen and take in some information, dismantle it, rearrange it, and integrate it into your life. Create. Play. Have fun with the process. Even if you only have a few seconds, that quieting of your mind is enough to ease access to your inner wisdom. Then let yourself make a choice. Choose what you want. Perhaps sometimes it's initially a small helping followed by a choice for seconds. Perhaps it's a large portion that you choose immediately and are not able to finish, or a smaller amount may be just right. Whatever choice you make, know that it is *your* choice—you are aware of it and embracing it because you are going to make the most of it, whatever it might be! Make the conscious decision to eat with the question "What eating experience do I want now?" Consider all the desires of body, mind, and soul and honor your decision.

Deciphering Mixed Messages

Desires to eat may present themselves to you with different degrees of urgency. You can consider their point and still make your decision. For example, if your body is telling you it is extremely hungry, it may be easy to let that desire take precedence over a certain taste of some kind and you will make a choice that will be satisfying and provide your body with the fuel that you need. A strong desire to eat for energy is likely to point you in a direction of a hearty sandwich or salad rather than a rich piece of chocolate. On the other hand, when you're feeling a desire for a comforting and satisfying treat to end a hard day that chocolate chip cookie may be just what you most desire. Perhaps you will have the experience of eating excessively when you hear your inner wisdom preferring to stop. Take in all that this moment offers, too. Don't let yourself label it as bad or out-of-control eating. Let it be.

Here are some other tips to consider when the answer to the question as to what eating experience you want now does not readily appear. If you are not sure where to begin, or listening to all the wants of your body, mind, and soul does not feel clear, then start by thinking about what your body may need. If you are hungry, but you don't feel much beyond that, then choose something nutritious and consistent with your health goals. Then if you realize what you want in the process do not try to talk yourself out of it. Eat what you really want. Be open to consider combining different foods to satisfy your entire self. For example, if you are in need of a substantial meal but only notice the craving for French fries, consider making food choices based on other nutritional needs to go along with your desire for French fries rather than choosing an entire meal of French fries. When you take all of your preferences into account you may find that smaller portions of specific tastes are more satisfying as a side dish than as an entire meal.

Pay attention to your *best self*'s changing needs and desires from moment to moment. You are making the decision only for right now. For example, perhaps you usually have pie at the pie shop. One evening you may not want pie. Habit suggests that you order a piece. Skip it and have pie on another day when that is what you really want. Similarly, a restaurant may have a Tuesday special that you usually enjoy. If, on a particular Tuesday, the special is not what you are hungry for, then don't order it. Have it on a Tuesday when you do want it. Recognize old habits and do not eat what you do not want. If you have yesterday's leftovers but do not want them, don't eat them. Since any food item is an option you will find that your *best self* will not choose to eat any food because "it might not have it again." Avoid common dieting behavior where food is eaten in large amounts to "get it out of the house" or because one is starting a program where they will never eat that food again. There is no longer any need to eat up all the ice cream because you are about to forbid it from entering the house. Perhaps your choices in eating may seem contradictory to the rule-bound thinking pattern. I know a couple that primarily buys their food from local, organic farm stands and eats very little processed food. This eating behavior is a part of who they are. Both of them make exceptions on vacation where they frequently stop at a fast-food ice cream chain with nonlocal, highly processed, nonorganic dairy treats that they thoroughly enjoy. Will they always do this? I don't know. It is what they choose now, without guilt.

The new information you have gathered regarding your food options and yourself also reside within you now. Don't be surprised if you begin to make some surprisingly different choices. For example, you may find that the craving for something refreshing and sweet might be met through a juicy slice of watermelon or a bunch of grapes or ice water with lemon rather than the double fudge ice cream cone that you have a personal history of eating on hot summer days. But if you decide it really is the double fudge ice cream cone that you want, then go ahead and enjoy it!

Personal Reflection

It was during an afternoon of shopping that I was able to observe the way that my *best self* was integrating my immediate need to eat with the information it was collecting about available food options. I discovered that I was hungry, but still had more to do before going home to eat so I asked myself, "What eating experience do I want now?" Since I wanted to finish the shopping I had set out to do and still get home in time to take my dogs for a walk before dark there was not time to eat a full meal. Delicious-looking assortments of candy bars were near the check out register. At first, my thoughts were focused on choosing which candy bar was my *best self* choice. Then, as I realized I wanted something with more nutritional substance than a candy bar offered, I explored other possibilities in my mind. I really wanted a snack that would give me substance and also satisfy my craving for something sweet that was triggered by the appealing row of candy bars I had just passed. The fast-food options available on my way to the next store held no appeal, neither did the apple in my car. I knew what I wanted to eat later in the evening and continued to explore options for my midday snack. When I saw a peanut butter and chocolate nutrition bar, I immediately knew that was what I wanted. It was the more satisfying version of the Butterfinger candy bar I had zeroed in on. This was my *best self* choice at that time. The bar was delicious and it gave me the energy I needed until I had time to make the dinner that I wanted at home.

Self-Reflections

In working with my clients, I have developed an exercise that many people find to be a helpful tool in increasing their faith in the intuitive process. Consider this exercise when you are choosing a favorite treat and answering the question, "What eating experience do I want now?" Here is an example of one person's response.

1. *What is your first choice to eat right now? What do you consider a satisfying portion of it to be?*

Food item: chocolate ice cream. **Satisfying portion:** 1 to 2 scoops

2. *What do you like about this favorite food?*

Food traits I like: I like the cold. I like the soft, soothing texture and I like the rich chocolate taste.

3. *How do you feel after you eat too much of this particular food?*

If I eat too much: I feel sluggish and have stomach cramps.

4. *What else might you really want when you are craving this food?*

Physically: Perhaps I want something sweet, something cold and refreshing to help coat my stomach after the spicy food I just had.

Emotionally: When I crave this food, I may want something to provide me comfort or something that I can nurture myself with. I may feel I deserve a treat. I might want to have some fun or just relax. Maybe I want something reminiscent of childhood fun. Perhaps I want to share something delicious with a friend.

5. *Allow yourself to eat a satisfying portion of this food. Consider how you feel. What needs does this food meet?*

Physically: I feel satisfied and comfortable. My stomach feels full. I am cooler in the hot weather and feel refreshed.

Emotionally: I enjoyed myself. But I still need to unwind from my busy day.

6. *Consider the possibility of having a second helping if you don't feel fulfilled, but allow a few minutes to distance yourself from your old patterns. Ask yourself, "Do I physi-*

cally need or want more food?" Then consider other options of things to eat or other non-eating things you might want to do.

Other foods that may be equally or more satisfying: Low-fat frozen yogurt, sorbet, fruit, a smoothie, or cold ice water with a lemon or lime slice, or bottled water.

7. If you still don't feel fulfilled, ask yourself questions like, "Am I emotionally hungry for something else? How might I respond to that need? What else might I want to do to satisfy my emotional need?" Try calling a friend, doing something fun, taking a bubble bath, playing with the dog, petting the cat, taking a nap, or listening to music.

Other things I like to do: Browse the internet, listen to music, watch a movie, throw the ball for my dog, sit outside, or call my nephew.

TAKE ACTION:
Determine Your Eating Experience

In order to keep your *best self* in the driver's seat, ask this question every time that you eat: What eating experience do I want now? Then before you eat, take a few minutes, or even just a few seconds if that is all that is available to you, and listen to what the needs and desires of your body, mind, and soul are at that moment. Then, in order to respond to these desires, think through the options that you have heard by listening to your inner wisdom. Having options available to you can make it easier to ward off SAD eating that has kept some hold on you.

The following ideas are not rules, they are suggestions based on the experiences of many who were transitioning from being SAD eaters to choosing from their *best selves*. Like any new information it is only meant for you to take in as it fits with your unique and natural relationship with food. Consider it more ammunition for removing the obstructing thought system of rule-based, outcome-focused dieting. They are possibilities that you can set up for yourself that encourage your body, mind, and soul to work together in choosing the eating experience that best fits the natural needs and desires of the current moment.

For your body:

Keep plenty of your top food choices available to you. These food choices should be aligned with your desire for eating experiences that promote your personal health and wellbeing. Consider having these options available to you in places like your home, in the car, at the office, or even in your purse or backpack. Do not starve your body. It's fine to feel hunger—some researchers say that waiting until you're hungry can even enhance healthy digestion—but do not keep your body in a deprived state for any period of time. Not only does it put your body into survival mode and reduce your metabolic rate, but it also sets you up for eating large amounts of food later on. This food may not be what you really want. If you feel yourself obsessing on body weight, choose a physical movement you enjoy to fight off any old SAD messages to alter your body though reduced eating.

For your mind:

Put the scale away. Better yet, give it away. It blocks the flow of your natural decision-making process by putting your focus back on losing weight. Wear comfortable clothes that fit you at the size you are right now. Buy new clothes that you consider attractive even if it is a size or two larger than you want to be. You need to feel comfortable without the reminder of clothing that is too tight. Consider getting a new hairstyle or color, or accessorize with glasses or jewelry, anything that might enhance your sense of physical presence that is unrelated to the size of your body.

For your soul:

With some of the time you spent in diet thoughts, do something for yourself. Relax, read, listen to music, or journal. Do something that comes easily or naturally for you, even if it is just for a few minutes at a time. This can help when restless thoughts about dieting find their way back into your mind. Consider practicing meditation where you can clear your mind. Remember you can choose to dismiss thoughts that may find their way into your brain. You are not obligated to address them, and can instead send them on their way. Replace them with peaceful and relaxing thoughts or mental images.

DAILY REMINDER:

I am free to choose my favorite food. When I honor my thoughts and feelings, I am able to fully enjoy the pleasurable qualities of my choices.

Deciding Not to Eat

Best self eating also means deciding not to eat. Sometimes the answer to the question "What eating experience do I want now?" is that you do not want to eat. So rather than it being a forced restriction you may choose not to eat when you realize that a food craving is actually showing you another need. The distracting thought that we want to eat may be covering up a deeper message from our innermost wisdom. Awareness that you do not really want to eat allows your inner voice to reveal your true need in the moment. For example, rather than eating more food to keep on going, you may need to take a break from what you are doing or go to bed. Your desire to get out of the office may reflect a need for fresh air rather than for a drive to the fast-food restaurant. The table on the following page illustrates common cravings that may be false food cravings suggesting a different *best self* option that does not involve eating.

True Craving	False Craving	Possible *Best Self* Option
Relaxation	Multiple doughnuts, a bag of candy, or large piece of frosted chocolate cake.	Take a bath, listen to music, sit outside, play with a pet, or read. Empty your mind.
Relief from tension	Bag of potato chips, fast food hopping, or overeating.	Take a walk or bike ride, dance, sing, talk to a friend, window shop, knit, or draw.
Relief from boredom	Picking at food all day long, opening the refrigerator multiple times, or eating with little satisfaction.	Volunteer, work on a personal project, talk to a friend, play, read, investigate a new hobby or a good cause, or learn something new.
Relief from loneliness	Lots of cookies, fast food hopping, or eating every few minutes with no satisfaction	Adopt a pet, do a random act of kindness, or spend time with family or friends.

Relief from exhaustion	Highly caffeinated drinks, candy bars, multiple cups of coffee, or wanting foods that you believe keep you awake.	Go to bed, take a nap, take a break, ask yourself why you are not allowing yourself a rest, or reduce the workload in your life.

TAKE ACTION:
Decode Your Cravings

Think of some of the common emotional cravings you experience that food does not truly satisfy. What non-eating activity would fulfill that true desire? Using the above table as a model, consider creating your own table so you can recognize the unique messages that your cravings have for you. So when you quiet your mind and ask, "What eating experience do I want now?" and listen deeply within, don't be surprised when the answer might be the realization that you want nothing. Rather than eat, think about what you might like to do instead. Try to choose an activity that will best fulfill your need.

DAILY REMINDER:
I trust my best self to consider the needs and desires of all of me when I ask the question, "What eating experience do I want now?" When I honor my thoughts and feelings I am able to fully enjoy the pleasurable qualities of what I choose to eat and decide not to eat.

CHAPTER V

STEP 5: EXPERIENCING

Celebrate Natural Eating Experiences

The fifth and last step on your way to discovering your natural relationship with food is fully embracing each and every eating experience. Now that a shift in your perspective has occurred, an entirely new approach to eating emerges. Eating is no longer an obsession, afterthought, or struggle. It is not an action that occurs when you fail to resist or control your desires. Eating is not simply a daily requirement or a fueling of the body for energy. So what is it, then? Eating is an experience to be treasured and always welcomed.

When I think about this final step on the journey to a new relationship with food the image of my dog Fritzi comes to mind. Fritzi danced with anticipatory joy and excitement for her food every day. The dance began as soon as she saw me get out her dish and ended when she took her first enthusiastic bite. After completing her meal, she gently leaped back to me as if to say, "Thanks." What kind of food experience will bring out a skip and a hop in you?

I believe that a spontaneous dance for joy originates from the soul. Freed from the restrictions of SAD, your *best self* now has the chance to allow food choices to come from your soul, your deepest essence. Soul is the place within you that has the capacity to bring unique meaning and joy to each life experience. Since most of us have to eat every day, usually a few times a day, food offers us a simple and continuous way to deepen that meaning and joy in our lives. Regardless of how busy you might be or how stressed you may feel with the demands and challenges of everyday life, when you ask yourself what eating experience you want at the present moment your inner wisdom invites soul and all of its vast possibilities into your everyday life.

Remember the Three As to *best self* eating? They guide each eating experience under the direction of the unique and natural relationship with food that is already within you. *Accepting* the moment at hand, your *authentic* or true desires have a chance to come together while your soul or innermost essence *appreciates* all that the eating experience has to offer. Freed from the limitations of SAD, food cravings and choices are a window to your soul and they can both reflect your innermost desires as well as provide ways to express your innermost feelings. Furthermore, your eating choices help you regain the ability to enhance the soulfulness in your life as they contribute to your other life experiences by adding old comforts and new joy, celebration, meaning, conviviality, and, let's not forget, an invaluable deeper connection with yourself.

The Eating Experience as a Window to Your Soul

When you no longer need to see cravings as impulses to ignore, you may discover that they offer insight into your deepest self. For example, I like to think that eating dog biscuits when I was young reflected my natural desire to understand and relate to my dog. I have heard that sometimes women who want to have a baby find themselves eating pickles, a craving that is often associated with being pregnant. Similarly, is a particular desire for chips and hot salsa that perhaps uncovers a need for more spice in one's life? Have you noticed that satisfying an urge for chocolate may sweeten an otherwise harsh kind of day? Struggles with food can take on new meaning when they are no longer judged and dismissed under SAD labels such as bad or overindulgent, or as a reflection of you having a lack of willpower. The following stories illustrate how soulful eaters gained insight into the inner workings of their souls through the conflicts they experienced in their food cravings:

> Joe began to crave a hot dog with mustard one particular afternoon. He usually preferred eating non-processed foods, such as whole grains, vegetables, and fruit. Because of his traditional eating preferences his craving for a hot dog surprised him. The more he ate his carrots and sprouts, the more he thought about his desire. After waking from a dream about hot dogs, he decided this mysterious food urge should not be ignored. Joe had fond memories of eating hot dogs smeared in mustard. He recalled going to baseball games with his brother when they were kids and "letting loose—shouting, laughing, and running around." They left their troubles behind as they climbed

the bleachers and feasted on ballpark franks. Lately, because Joe had been working so hard to finish a project at work, he had not had much time to spend with his family. Was his inner voice trying to say something through this unusual food craving? Joe concluded that his desire for a hot dog might be telling him that he needed to spend more time with his family, perhaps specifically with his brother. How did Joe answer this message? He explored ways to satisfy both his craving and his emotional need. Initially, he took a short break from work and took a walk with his son to a nearby hot dog stand. He also planned to get tickets to a ball game to celebrate his brother's upcoming birthday. When he did not deny this specific food craving, he received the deeper message about what he needed and was willing to explore its significance in his life. With a new awareness of the impact his busy work life was having on himself and his family, Joe was able to explore choices that enriched both his eating and living experiences.

Mary's battle with a cookie craving shows another way eating desires offer a deeper self-understanding. Mary had a long diet history and was developing her own personal approach to food when she relayed to me a valuable lesson she had learned. Her insight occurred while studying for a college final. With only an hour remaining before the exam, she was trying to cram pages of notes into her mind, but was distracted by a strong urge for chocolate chip cookies. She knew she was a little nervous, but did not accept that as an explanation for her sudden obsession. She explored the possible meaning of this craving by writing in her journal. The following is an excerpt from her writing that day:

I am nervous because I really did not study enough. I would prefer being more prepared. Whether I eat the cookies or not, I know next time I will be more prepared. Maybe I am nervous because doing well on this test is something I truly value. I deeply want to succeed. I have been studying so hard to meet this goal that I have not given myself enough nurturing along the way, so I'm craving something for me—a cookie craving. I want to reconsider how long I need to sacrifice nurturing myself to achieve what I want. Maybe there is a little more room for compromising.

Once she could acknowledge and allow a clearer understanding of her eating impulse, Mary could decide what to do about this persistent desire. She put her book away, took a few deep breaths, and, since she did not have enough time just then to go out and buy cookies, she enjoyed a cup of hot chocolate from a machine in a nearby student lobby. She enjoyed the distraction and felt nurtured. She decided to plan to visit a friend after the test, rent a movie, choose some favorite foods to eat, and, most importantly, make a trip to the local bakery to pick up some chocolate chip cookies.

In addition to revealing our soul's wishes, there are simple ways that we can choose to express our genuine selves, with even the simplest consideration of preferences. I have a collection of assorted coffee mugs. I consciously choose one with colors, a design, or association that goes along with my mood each morning. Some are brightly colored and others have pictures of dogs, cats, birds, and angels on them. I associate some of the cups with places I have traveled and others remind me of friends with whom I have shared a cup of tea.

People have told me that they find eating crunchy food like carrots or pretzels to be good tension releasers. Just like hitting a pillow, frustration can find a physical expression in eating corn on the cob and biting into a hard and crisp chilled apple. Others find that they can satisfy their need for creativity after completing a tedious task like tax preparation by experimenting with unusual food combinations and concoctions. Don't be afraid to find expression of your feelings through food experiences. Why not? There are so many natural chances everyday to let food bring out your feelings. Experiment with the unique food experiences that best express your feelings.

Uncovering the Simple Pleasures of Eating

With SAD thinking no longer at the forefront of your mind, you realize that your desire for food is natural and not something to fight or a reason for feeling guilty. The energy that you will use to live your day comes from the fuel that you give to your body in response to its request for food. By accepting your body's messages of hunger as a reflection of your desire to be alive, just the basic pleasure that comes from giving your body the nourishment it needs becomes available to you.

The pleasure goes even further, however, because we are not simply responding to our need for fuel. Rather, we are exploring what eating experience we desire beyond the physical need of the body. Simple pleasures abound and include comforts, connectedness with others, and an invitation to unlimited adventures and possibilities.

Experiencing the Comforts of Food

Depending on how we choose to use food, it can provide daily comfort as a constant in our lives. Eating gives us a break from our work. It offers a distraction from our thoughts. Most of us find the need for self-soothing at different times in our lives and would agree that food can sometimes offer that comfort. A specific food's ability to console may be derived from a memory, an association, a texture, a pleasant social experience, or can occur for an unexplainable reason.

Understanding your unique comfort foods gives you the chance to design eating experiences that offer that extra little joy when you need it. You may have a particular association of comfort with a very specific food; however, there also are many examples of foods that inherently seem to hold universal comforting appeal such as a juicy piece of fruit, freshly baked bread, and a warm piece of fruit pie *a la mode*. While sometimes you may want the exact food that created the association with comfort in the first place, you may also understand the characteristics of the food that bring the pleasure and create even better ones! For example, the fun teenage experience of eating potato chips and dip with your pals might be made more enjoyable as a health-conscious adult by sharing crunchy raw vegetables and hummus with friends. The pleasure previously derived from a candy bar may now be satisfied with a delicious, juicy orange.

A perfect example of honoring the memories of childhood eating experiences with the changing preferences one might have as an adult is the creative solution that my vegan niece Laura discovered on her annual family vacation to a cabin on a lake. Part of the experience every year, from the age of one through her current age of twenty-five, has been a family outing in a boat to a little ice cream shop. They each choose from a delicious array of flavors that are always different than the year before, and everyone enjoys an ice cream cone before getting back on the boat. When Laura first became vegan she chose not to have the ice cream cone, but asked if the manager might consider purchasing a vegan option. She reported feeling like she was deprived as she watched her siblings enjoy the annual tradition of the ice cream cone. The following year she discovered that a refreshing non-dairy "ice cream" treat option was still not available. She instead purchased a snack that really did not "hit the spot" and she once again felt deprived as her family enjoyed their annual ice cream treats. Last year she decided to pack up a pint of her favorite vegan nondairy dessert in a cooler and she brought it on the boat along with a serving spoon. She bought a cone at the ice cream shop, put her own nondairy dessert in it, and enjoyed eating her treat along with her family while also honoring her preference to be vegan. With no feeling of deprivation, she also noticed how much easier it felt to digest her option and enjoyed that extra benefit, too. A similar experience occurs for me when I chose not to eat meat. Although I have many fond memories throughout my childhood of sharing my dad's favorite lunch of hamburger and fries, my present choice to not eat meat overrides any pleasurable association I have about eating meat. It holds no appeal to me and feels like a *best self* choice and in no way a restriction.

Many others have reported this experience to me of altering the particular food they choose to eat while at the same time reminiscing about food they especially enjoyed as a child. Some of us grew up enjoying chocolate cupcakes with the rubbery coating of frosting or the bright yellow oblong cakes with the white glob inside wrapped in a cellophane package (I won't mention any brand names). While there may be some comforting associations attached to these childhood snacks, a healthier, less processed and packaged substitute may be more satisfying and easier to digest and still offer the same pleasurable nostalgic feeling. The point is that when you need the comfort of food, go ahead and have it in whatever old or new form it may take for you. Trust your *best self* to consider the comfort of food as it creates your unique experience.

Personal Reflection

My husband and I enjoy his mother's exquisite spaghetti sauce. To accommodate our desire for a vegan version, she revised an original recipe that has been passed on through multiple generations of nurturing Italian mothers. In the summertime, the sauce would take on new flavors and textures as my husband's father added his homegrown sweet red peppers, tomatoes, and fresh basil. My in-laws' love was felt in every bite, and my husband enjoyed the flavors reminiscent of childhood dinners and family gatherings.

Finally, in addition to providing comfort in the moment, the anticipation of an upcoming enjoyable eating experience can help get you through a more challenging present moment. What special treat might you look forward to at the end of a hard day? I receive much more pleasure while removing winter snow from my driveway when I keep in mind the image of the cup of hot chocolate I will have when I am finished. An oil change for my car feels like a less tedious task when I think about a favorite restaurant nearby where I will eat while I am waiting. How can you enhance the present moment with the thought of a favorite food at the completion a task?

Personal Reflection

For many years now, my friend Vicki and her daughter Rocio help me thoroughly clean my house every month. It's an all day event and the highlight for all of us is the time we set aside for lunch. Sometimes the meal is my own creation and other times Vicki and Rocio prepare food for me to experience. Lunch feels like a much-deserved break in our day and is a greatly anticipated delight that we share together at the kitchen table. Table conversations may have included discussions that bring laughter or tears, intriguing stories, and even problem solving when needed.

Experiencing Connectedness with Others through Food

In addition to the option of choosing a specific food that brings us comfort, another attribute of food is its continued ability to remind of us of the meaningful and joyful times with others. Foods and drinks seem designed to be part of our sense of connectedness with people—past, present, and future. It reminds us of the experiences we had, it adds to the ones we are having, and it becomes part of the anticipated pleasure in experiences to come. As you welcome food as an integral part of your life's journey, the soul is given the chance to enhance life's joy and meaning as it presents itself in the significant happenings in your lives. Food is typically present in both the joyful celebrations, such as weddings and graduations, as well as the gatherings that are associated with more challenging times, such as wakes or funerals. Think of all the special occasions that are more fully enjoyed with the food spreads, the appetizers, the barbeque grills, and the scrumptious cake and desserts. The sharing of traditional foods and rituals around these events as well as unique favorite choices are designed to bring meaning and fuller pleasure to the event.

With its soulful qualities, food experiences enhance our sense of relatedness with others. When food is present, the soul can enter even the most ordinary conversation with a friend or business meeting. It has always seemed to me that problems were easier to solve while sipping coffee on the back porch or while being served a delicious breakfast in a cozy restaurant. When a friend brings a favorite food to another friend in need or when a mother cooks her child's favorite meal on a weekend visit from college the giver's expression of love is likely to add to the meal's enjoyment. The opportunity to share good food with others while supporting a cause close to one's heart certainly adds to the appeal of a community fundraiser or benefit. Neighbors express their care for each other by preparing homemade meals and bringing them to their homes in times of crisis.

Personal Reflection

Sometimes comfort and connectedness are both part of the meaningful eating experience. I recall a time when my sister came to town and she and I both enjoyed a new refreshing lime drink from a coffee shop. A few weeks after she returned to Minnesota I made my own more natural version of the fruit drink at home and enjoyed the refreshment as well as its ability to take me back to the fun I had spending time with my sister. There are also certain snacks that my great nephews and I usually enjoy together when they visit, especially those that we eat after a hard day of play. The food we choose adds to the fun and adventure of our time together. After they return home, I am able to recapture their joyful spirits and reminisce about our time together by eating the same treats.

Experiencing New and Unexpected Opportunities from Food

Your *best self* is eager to create an eating experience from any situation with food that it is given. An interaction with food that fulfills your body, mind, and soul is a good start, but adding a little unexpected pleasure, insight, or mystery to the experience is even better! As the following story illustrates, even in the most unlikely situation an opportunity to create a meaningful eating experience may present itself to us and it is ours for the taking, adding pleasure and even a little mystery to our everyday lives:

> While vacationing in Italy, a couple was involved in a minor car accident. Although relieved that no one was hurt, they were tired, hungry, and upset because the day would be lost. The driver of the other car involved in the accident was a sixty-year-old, English speaking, native Italian man. He confirmed the couple's fear that

the police would probably not arrive for hours and proposed that they have lunch together. Following his suggestion, they walked down the block to a quaint garden café. They were seated in the sun among colorful and aromatic flowers where Italian music, voices, and laughter filled the air. They recalled that they had the best pasta, fresh bread, wine, and conversation they have ever had. The couple learned more about Italy in that afternoon than they had during the previous three days. The couple knew they had shared an experience that would dwell deep within their souls.

Experiencing New and Unexpected Opportunities in the Old Ways from Food

It is easy to forget that the enjoyment we receive in sharing food experiences with others is equally available to us when we are eating alone. Consider the opportunity to create new ways of experiencing eating by yourself. So many times I have heard people say, "I am not going to bother to cook anything when it is just for me." My response is usually "Why not?" As a matter of fact, it offers the unique opportunity for you to completely focus on creating the experience exactly to your liking, with no need to consider anyone else. Consider your options. If you really prefer a quick peanut butter and jelly sandwich, then don't let me stop you. On the other hand, if you enjoy cooking or baking and have something in mind that you would like to make and eat, but are reluctant because it's "just for you," go ahead and try it. If the recipe you use makes too much, only use half the amount of ingredients, or make it all and freeze it for another day. You can always give away extra baked goods to friends, family, coworkers, or neighbors. Perhaps you are feeling lonely wishing there was someone with whom you could share a meal. That might be just the time to become distracted with preparing yourself a nurturing dinner completely suited to your tastes and preferences. Take advantage of the fact that you only need to focus on what *you* want and nobody else. You can experiment and try something new. The same goes for eating outside your home. Just because it's just you for dinner doesn't mean you can only get carryout at a fast-food drive-through. You can still choose to sit down and eat at a restaurant of your choice. You can take yourself out on a picnic. Or you can get carryout food and set up a place at the table for you to leisurely nurture yourself with a placemat and the same plates and trimmings that you would have when eating with others. Remember that as you allow your *best self* to take charge of your new eating experiences, none of the old rules apply. Allow yourself to see all the options that are available as you welcome new eating experiences.

Experiencing New and Unexpected Opportunities Now from Food

No longer focused on the SAD thoughts that obstruct our joy in the moment (e.g. what we should not have eaten in the past and what we will try not to eat in the future), we are free to truly consider what we want *right now*. Not only does eating become more pleasurable, it also enhances the soulfulness in our lives by allowing us to spend more time in the present. We can bring ourselves fully back to the present by involving all of our senses in the creation of the eating experience. We can enhance the enjoyment of our interactions with food by involving the desires of the five senses—touch, smell, taste, sight, and sound—in creating and enjoying the eating experiences that are present.

Touch: Think about your texture preferences when you choose, prepare, and eat food. What appeals to you? Soft, crispy, juicy, dry, or chewy? Notice how your choice in eating utensil also creates different sensations. For example, bringing my own cup when I travel indulges my preference for the feel of ceramic over a Styrofoam or paper cup on my lips and in my hands when enjoying coffee. How can you enhance your unique eating experiences through touch?

Smell: When it comes to eating the smell of food can stimulate many pleasant associations while preparing, cooking, and eating. Other fragrances that become part of the experience can also enhance the pleasure in the moment. Outdoor eating might involve the smell of flowers, food cooking on a grill, or simply the delight of taking in a breath of fresh air. What aromas are particularly enjoyable for you?

Taste: Take a moment to savor the flavor in your mouth. Would you like to add a slice of lemon or lime to your glass of water? Consider adding another spice to your slice of pizza or side of vegetables. Honor your desire for a mint or something sweet after your meal and then delight in all the pleasurable sensations that it offers. What specific tastes can you take pleasure in the next time you choose to eat?

Sight: In addition to enjoying how attractive your food can be, pay attention to the visual atmosphere. For example, create a scene for yourself if you are home alone and planning to eat. Think about what visually enhancing ways you can improve the moment with. What would a table cloth, certain dishes, lighting a candle, or sitting by a window with a view add to your eating experience?

Sound: Sounds created by preparing and cooking food may hold certain appeal. For me, listening to popcorn pop and vegetables in a wok sizzle are part of the pleasure of those two foods. Other ways that sound can enhance an eating atmosphere might include playing music, finding a quiet place, or eating while listening to the radio. You can enhance the joy of a celebration with food by taking in the noises around you: laughing, talking, and perhaps even the moving and clanging of plates and eating utensils at the event. What sounds can you include in your next eating experience to enhance the mood you want to create?

When you allow all of your senses to contribute to the moment you not only appreciate your food more, but your time spent in the present enhances your enjoyment of life.

TAKE ACTION:
Embrace the Eating Experiences in Your Life

To help embrace the joys in the moment, consider the following questions when creating even the simplest everyday eating experience.

Touch

- What textures of food appeal to me?
- How do I like to touch my food? What kinds of eating utensils do I like? Do I like to eat with my fingers? Do I prefer to bite into an apple or cut it up?

Smell

- What past associations do I have with certain smells?
- What are my favorite food aromas?
- What are some foods I may want to cook to put more fragrance into my life?

Taste

- How can I increase my awareness of taste?
- Do I need to slow my eating pace to enjoy the taste?
- What tastes do I like to combine? What little things can I add to my food to satisfy my taste preferences?

Sight

- What do I like to see while I eat?
- What are some of my favorite places to eat because of the attractive atmosphere?
- How can I create a visually appealing atmosphere for eating at work?

- How can I do the same at home?

Sound

- What kind of music adds to my eating experience?
- What sounds do I enjoy in the restaurants I choose?
- What do I like to hear while preparing food?

Personal Reflection

As I conclude this chapter on celebrating eating experiences in the now, I want to provide an illustration of the coming together of authenticity, acceptance, and appreciation in one of my recent ordinary yet thoroughly enjoyable and meaningful connections with food. Below is my account of the eating experience as it unfolded:

> While revising this chapter, I felt hungry. It didn't really matter to me when I ate last or how much I have eaten today. I responded to my immediate feelings of hunger and need for a break. So I asked myself, "What eating experience do I want now?" Since I have been asking myself this question for many years now, multiple times a day, it has become second nature for me to intuitively arrive at an answer quite quickly. A quick review of the moment told me that I knew that I wanted to take only a short break from writing, I would be eating alone, and I preferred not to leave the house. A broccoli sandwich was my immediate first choice; that is, until I realized I had cooked the last of it in a rice and veggie stir fry I had prepared for my husband to take with him to work that day. As I browsed the

refrigerator, I noticed a pack of shredded cabbage and carrots as well as a package of shredded broccoli and carrots. I knew right then what I wanted. So in one of my new orange and yellow ceramic bowls with a daisy design, I mixed up a batch of coleslaw to my liking, adding frozen peas, celery, dressing, salt, and pepper. I completely enjoyed everything about this eating experience and I felt satisfied as I continued writing. It then occurred to me that perhaps dissecting and writing about this spontaneous eating experience of mine might be a way to describe soulful eating, so I immediately wrote the following:

I have no idea how many calories or grams of fat my snack contained. I enjoyed fixing it. I like the new bowl I bought. It makes me feel happy. I have always loved mixing textures and colors together. Frozen peas were a favorite food of mine from childhood. The taste of the vinaigrette reminded me of a meal I had with my family the Friday after Thanksgiving last year when I was introduced to this particular dressing. While eating the coleslaw, I found my mind reminiscing about that meal and smiling as I thought about my three- and five-year-old great nephews who were at the gathering. I also had several flashbacks of eating frozen peas out of the bag as a child. The coleslaw was delicious; I enjoyed the crunching textures and sounds, the fresh tastes, and noticed the visual appeal of the various colors in the bright orange bowl. I have returned to writing, completely satisfied; I thoroughly enjoyed my break. My body received good nourishment. And until I asked the question, "What eating experience do I want now," I had no pre-planned meal on my mind. My soul presented itself throughout the eating experience: my happy and colorful bowl, the fond memories the meal triggered, and the spontaneity and creativity of my meal. All my senses were awakened with the textures, colors, smells, and tastes. With an energized body, mind, and soul, I enthusiastically returned to my task at hand.

Self-Reflections

Look back on your food struggles. Can you see ways that they reflect your life struggles?

- What are your comfort foods? Why? When do you need them most?

- What foods bring you warm feelings and good memories?

- What ways do you most enjoy sharing food experiences with others?

- How open can you be to spontaneous experiences with food?

- What can you celebrate with food today?

Beyond Eating

Your *best self* is now activated, energized, and empowered as it guides you to new experiences with food. It can't be stopped and you wouldn't want it to be. With SAD thinking no longer an influence, your inner wisdom enjoys the path that has been cleared as it creates eating experiences aligned with your natural *best self*. You have experienced the freedom that happens when you dismantle a thought system that you had come to believe and eat by. The obstructing thoughts that block your ability to hear the voice of your soul are gone. You are no longer controlled by the misdirected thoughts about eating patterns of the past. You are no longer making decisions based on expectations for an outcome of weight loss. Your present actions come from fully taking in all that the present moment has to offer when you listen deeply within. You are ready to soar in all directions that you allow your *best self* to go and there are unlimited possibilities. And each fulfilling eating experience only strengthens its position as director in your life.

So if you can so easily change your relationship with food, what else might you uncover if you let your *best self* continue this same path in other areas of your life? Open that door to these endless possibilities. Look how the rediscovery of your natural relationship with food lights the way for you to choose to live more fully in all aspects of your everyday life. You now know that you can:

1) question and let go of any thoughts blocking your ability to listen to your inner wisdom

2) make choices that integrate the needs and desires of all of you—body, mind, and soul

3) trust your own intuitive understanding

4) find all that you need is in the present moment at hand

5) discover the gifts of insight, expression, mystery, joy, and meaning in everyday experiences

6) choose what you want to know and what you do with the information you gain

7) let your inner wisdom guide you in any way you choose—it already knows what to do

Now take what you have discovered beyond your relationship with food and fully embrace each and every experience as you step into the fresh possibilities that life offers.

SELF-AFFIRMATIONS FOR *BEST SELF* EATING AND LIVING

For many ex-dieters, understanding the concepts of giving up SAD gives them the strength and tools to master the techniques used in *best self* eating. Others find that having specific statements to say to themselves, or to display as visual reminders of their new approach to eating, are invaluable. The following is a list of self-affirmations that I have compiled based on my experiences with clients' needs as they made the transition from SAD eating to soulful, *best self* eating. You may want to choose a few that appeal to you and say them to yourself every morning before you begin your day. Some may be particularly helpful when you find yourself battling a thought from the mindset of rule-bound eating. The following self-affirmations are designed to strengthen your commitment to trusting your inner wisdom.

Self-Affirmations for Uncovering the Obstructing Thoughts of Rule-bound Eating

- I am in charge of exploring my options regarding what, when, and where I choose to eat. I can choose to eat whatever, whenever, and wherever I want.

- Given the information I have about food, I can trust my own food choices.

143

- If I choose a food that causes me physical discomfort, I will consider that reaction before making that choice again.

- I will remind myself that I am free to eat any way I choose.

- I am free to consider any food item.

- I am free to reject any food item.

- I will not allow myself to give in to the urge to "forbid" a food, or a time or a place to eat.

- I am free to choose not to eat at times and places prescribed by previous diets.

- I now replace "bad" eating days with learning days. I will not put myself down for having a day I think of as bad eating because I will gain an opportunity to learn about myself.

- I will not let a diet system control my feeling of self-worth.

- I will not waste my time and energy dieting.

- I will discover my natural eating patterns by exploring my eating behavior rather than condemning it.

- I can make different food choices daily and allow my eating experiences to vary from day to day.

Self-Affirmations for Allowing Your *Best Self* the Freedom of Choice

- I will allow myself to become aware of what I *really* want to eat.

- I will enjoy the satisfied feeling of eating what I really want.

- If I really want to eat something that is not readily available to me, I can go ahead and get it instead of settling for a substitute.

- I will become aware of what it feels like to eat what I *really* want as opposed to eating what I think I should.

- If what I really want is not available, I can eat nothing. I can decide to wait and eat what I want later.

- I am prepared to experience some unusual eating episodes until my tastes and cravings become fully integrated into my own natural process of eating.

- I can choose to engage in physical activities that

truly appeal to me for reasons other than to burn calories or fat.

- I will give up structured exercise programs designed strictly to burn calories or fat.

- I will explore physical activities that I like and do them when I want to do them.

Self-Affirmations to Choose the Identity of a *Best Self* Eater

- I am no longer limited by dieting.

- I am proud that I am not a dieter.

- I am proud to have overcome SAD eating.

- Rule-bound eating for weight loss is no longer a part of me.

- I will not allow weight loss rules concerning my eating habits determine my self-worth.

- Dieting is the wrong approach to solving life's problems. It suppresses my true ability to deal with difficult situations.

- I will not give in to the urge to diet. There are NO

good reasons to diet for the sole purpose of weight loss.

- I accept my freedom to structure my life in my own way, not according to the demands of a diet.

- My ultimate goal is to achieve a relationship with food that is peacefully integrated into my daily life.

- It is natural for me to feel anxiety about letting go of everything I learned about dieting, but I will continue to allow my *best self* to direct my choices.

- I can eat to enhance my enjoyment of an experience.

- I can eat when I am feeling sad or happy.

- I can eat to celebrate.

- I can decide to eat in order to relax when I am nervous.

- Food is more than just fuel for the body.

- I will allow emotional eating to help uncover and express feelings.

- It is a gift to be able to use food as an emotional outlet.

- I am willing to fight the social pressures to diet.

- I will eat for fun.

More Self-Affirmations for Integrating *Best Self* Eating and Living

- I will recognize my freedom of choice to live my life without hiding behind dieting.

- I will trust myself to make healthy food choices that consider my body, mind, and soul.

- I am open to listening to my true needs.

- I am open to accepting all of me, both my strengths and my weaknesses.

- I will strive to face others and myself with authenticity, acceptance, and appreciation.

- I will continue to search deep inside myself to find the answers held within.

- I will allow myself to have satisfying eating experiences.

- I will replace the goal of weight loss with the goal of a natural relationship with food under the direction of my *best self.*

- I will continue to become informed about my food choices and myself, not programmed.

- I will look at my eating experiences as a window to expressions of some of my deepest needs and desires.

CONCLUSION

This is not the end, but rather the beginning of a new journey with the life-enriching relationship with food that has always been within you. If this book has done its job, your *best self* is bubbling over with excitement as it reclaims its natural role as director of your everyday eating experiences. Did you notice yourself filling in the empty spaces of this interactive guide with your own inner wisdom? As you uncover your natural and ever-changing relationship with food—one eating experience at a time— you will continue to enhance your life as you continue to give your natural relationship with food its life.

Eat! Begin your journey on the path back to a fulfilling, healthy, and real relationship with your food— *your* relationship with food. Open the door to unlimited possibilities in your life, but first take a moment and quiet your mind. Ask yourself, "What eating experience do I want now?" Listen fully and deeply to the voice of your *best self*. You will know what to do—you always have and you always will. Now eat, live, and enjoy!

Afterword by the Author

As I complete this book, I am drawn to reflecting back on the changing nature of my relationship with food during these past sixteen years since the *Tao of Eating* (Innisfree, 1998), my previous book, was first published. Integrated into my everyday life, my eating experiences continue to reveal and enhance my authentic life's journey. Realizing that self-nurturing includes much more than just food, *Give to Your Heart's Content . . . without Giving Yourself Away* was first published in 2002 by Innisfree Press and then again in 2004 by InnerOcean Publishing, after it was revised and re-released. I have continued to work in my clinical practice along with my husband for the past thirty years.

Consistent with my love of animals and new understanding of the relationship between humans and animals, my eating choices are always vegetarian, primarily vegan. I try to make food choices that do not involve the suffering of animals. While this way of eating eliminates many foods, I do not experience it as restrictive. For me, it is freeing and self-affirming, consistent with the authentic beliefs and desires of my innermost self. I enjoy choosing, making, creating, cooking, and eating food more than I ever have. My eating experiences nurture my body, mind, and soul. They support and reflect my current life's journey, which includes the recent writing of my book titled *The Power of Joy in Giving to Animals,* enhancing my authentic relationships with humans and animals. My daily work and activities feed my soul just as my eating experiences feed my soul and truly reflect its inner workings. Eating experiences enhance the soulfulness in my life, while my soul enhances my eating experiences.

ABOUT THE AUTHOR

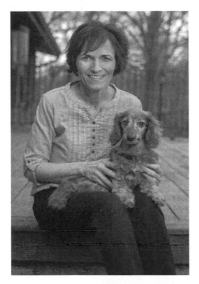

Photo by Adriana Acevedo

Linda R. Harper, Ph.D., is a licensed clinical psychologist in private practice for over thirty years with her husband in the Chicago area. She is an international speaker and offers workshops, talks, and individual consults on a variety of topics related to self-care for the body, mind, and soul. Her current practice is designed to help people uncover their natural inner wisdom so they can fully embrace and experience all that life has to offer to them and all that their unique gifts have to offer to life.

Dr. Harper's latest book is *The Power of Joy in Giving to Animals*. She is also the author of *The Tao of Eating: Feeding Your Soul through Everyday Experiences with Food, Give to Your Heart's Content . . . without Giving Yourself Away, Eat: A Guide to Discovering Your Natural Relationship with Food*, and *Give: A Guide to Discovering the Joy of Everyday Giving*.

For more, visit www.harperhelper.com